PREFACE

My first words to you in this book are that if you are suffering from GERD (or GORD as it's known here in the UK) - what you're going through is real and it matters.

I say that because so often when you experience a health problem, especially when it's so chronic, nobody really stops to acknowledge just how much it can affect that person. In the case of GERD, it's exhausting not to be able to eat properly, being constantly afraid to try and eat and then suffering the consequences when you try and eat something slightly different to what you've been able to eat up to now. Add on any other health problems into the mix, and it's even more draining. So take the time to recognise your experience is valid, and no you shouldn't have to just live with it.

Now, if someone was to tell you that experiencing GERD actually presents a golden opportunity to change your life for the better, you'd probably suspect they had pasted one of those inheritance email scams into their book draft by mistake. Only, there is some truth that you will gain riches in terms of your health (which ironically, money cannot buy!) and that you are royalty to yourself because there is only one of you.

What I mean here is that GERD is your body's way of telling you that it's not working optimally. It wants you to fix the underlying issue so that it can work to the best of its ability. So, are you finally going to listen, or are you going to discard all of these warning signs like you do indeed those scam emails? Only, there's no con to healing from GERD - this really is a chance to change your life for the better, since we cannot function properly if our gut is out of whack. I can guarantee every aspect of your life will soon become affected if it hasn't already if you have chronic GERD.

As I will stress throughout, I'm not a doctor and I'm certainly no replacement for informed medical care. I am however, someone who suffered from GERD quite severely for a period of around 18 months. I was put on all the different medications you probably have been and went through a rigmarole of different scans, doctors and even hospitals. In the end, I was able to recover through my own interventions.

I will state none of what I did is anything I think any doctor would take issue with. The reason I am writing this book is that the information simply isn't out there. Even when I referred to a specialist to see if there was any intervention they could take - at no time was a diet plan or healing strategy mentioned. I was left to figure it out on my own when I have zero medical training. I don't understand why this is the case when GERD is an extremely common problem.

We know our doctors and nurses do incredible work, but in the case of GERD, there's simply not enough information for patients to be able to create an actual plan to move forward. After all, when it comes to eating, this is something a healthy person does several times a day without even thinking about it. But when you're suffering from severe GERD it's 24/7. You become extremely restricted with the food and drink you can consume. Even sipping the wrong tea can leave you in agony for days. Yet, you still have to go to work, pay the bills, take care of the kids and carry on with any other responsibilities you might have as an adult. How are people supposed to do all that when they can barely swallow a mouthful of food without feeling as if there is a blowtorch in their stomach? A specialist I spoke to actually shrugged his shoulders when I raised that point.

I originally posted a video about my GERD struggles over on my YouTube channel. My channel is only small, as it's just a hobby I do outside of my actual work. So imagine my surprise when the video hits 200,000 views and what feels like the same amount of messages to every inbox I have, with people all going through the exact same thing as me. Like, what on earth?! I knew that I wouldn't be able to answer each person to the level they needed, hence a book will give you all the answers and hopefully more. I want to give you an actual strategy to heal and recover from this horrific illness.

I think it's important for patients to speak up, especially if they have found a positive resolution to any condition. That's because so often, you only find people struggling. You rarely find people who report back and help guide those who were once in their position. I believe if more people did this (again, without trying to replace that person's doctor), then maybe more people could feel both reassurance and relief. It's a way of giving back that can add so much value to someone else who was once in your shoes.

Really important disclaimer: I want you to maintain a good relationship with your doctor, yes even if you feel frustrated. At the end of the day, they are the only ones who can prod you, scan you and prescribe any medication to you. No author, even if they themselves are a doctor (which I'm not), can do this. Therefore, it's so important you read my book but in tandem with seeking proper medical care. I genuinely want each person to get better because GERD is a very lonely and difficult condition to experience. So, think of me as someone you met in the waiting room at your doctor's office, rather than me being the actual doctor, which I'm not and very few people actually are. As stated, I am a patient who has been through GERD, and what I have written in this book is the steps I took to recover, along with a broader view of the condition and why I think it's become so incredibly common in today's society.

I can't believe I'm writing this, but I also have to point out it's not enough to just buy this book alone - you have to actually make every effort to listen and follow what's in it. On my video comments, I had a lot of people asking me to 'help them', instead of listening to what I was saying and going away and doing it. You can lead a horse to water, but you can't make it drink as they say. Well, I need you to dig deep and take a big gulp here, because your healing is now in your own hands.

It's time to take responsibility for your own health, to make changes that are actually going to help you feel better for the rest of your life, especially if your GERD is diet or lifestyle related. If you're at the stage where you are buying books because nothing else has worked, I think you're ready. So let's begin.

Editor's note: This book has been written in British English as the author is from the UK, but some common medical terms will be written in American English (i.e. 'esophagus' rather than 'oesophagus') to try to ensure clarity for as many different audiences as possible.

CONTENTS

Preface
Dedication
Title Page
1.0 What Is GERD?   1
1.1 GERD Symptoms   5
1.2 What Causes GERD?   7
1.3 Heartburn Vs GERD   18
1.4 My GERD Story   21
1.5 My GERD Recovery   58
1.6 Getting GERD Diagnosed   64
1.7 GERD: Why There's No Easy Way Out   67
1.8 Preparing Yourself For Change   70
1.9 Dealing With Hopelessness   74
2.0 My Experience With GERD Medication   78
2.1 The Pink Goo   84
2.2 My Thoughts On Apple Cider Vinegar   87
3.0 Eating With GERD   89
3.1 The pH Scale Explained   92
3.2 What Not To Eat With GERD   108
3.3 What Not To Drink With GERD   114

3.4 Ditching The SAD Diet	118
3.5 Mindful Eating	123
3.6 What To Do If You're Struggling To Eat	126
3.7 Eating Top Tips	128
4.0 GERD Recovery Diet Plan	131
4.1 Breakfast	137
4.2 Lunch	145
4.3 Dinner	150
4.4 Snacks	155
4.5 Additional Supplements	158
4.6 Camomile Tea	160
4.7 Probiotics	164
4.8 Reintroducing Foods	171
4.9 Bringing A GERD Flare Under Control	174
5.0 Stress	177
5.1 Recognising You're Stressed	185
5.2 Toxic Environments	187
5.3 Work Stress	190
5.4 Digital Stress	200
5.5 Societal Pressure	202
5.6 The Wrong Ways To Deal With Stress	204
5.7 The Right Ways To Deal With Stress	208
6.0 Lifestyle	211
6.1 Exercising With GERD	212
6.2 Sleeping With GERD	214
6.3 Travelling With GERD	217
6.4 Eating Out With GERD	223
6.5 Pregnancy And GERD	226

6.6 Posture And GERD	229
6.7 Lifestyle Top Tips	230
7.0 The Post GERD Years	234
7.1 What I Would Have Told Myself	236
7.2 What I Want Healthcare Professionals To Know	237
8.0 Conclusion	239
8.1 GERD FAQ	243
8.2 GERD Be Gone	248
About The Author	249

Thank you to my mother Sharon, and my partner Isaak for supporting me through my GERD journey.

I'll never win an Oscar so that was my acceptance speech bit. As you were.

HOW I RECOVERED FROM GERD - A PATIENT'S PERSPECTIVE

The Rachael Edit

1.0 WHAT IS GERD?

GERD stands for gastroesophageal reflux disease, aka **G**astro**E**sophageal **R**eflux **D**isease.

It is estimated that 20% of Americans have GERD at any one time, which equates to approximately 66 million people in the USA alone. Per continent, it is thought that between 8.8% and 33.1% of the population are suffering from GERD. In total, this amounts to millions of people all around the world experiencing these same debilitating symptoms as you. So no, you are certainly not alone, and yes, GERD is very much an epidemic that we need to work harder to solve.

For the uninitiated, GERD is a disorder whereby your stomach acid flows up into the esophagus (oesophagus in British English), which is the tube connecting your mouth to your stomach. The most basic way of explaining why that's a problem is because your stomach acid is not designed to be anywhere other than your stomach.

Usually, a valve called the lower esophageal sphincter (LES) keeps your stomach acid contained. However, the LES can become weakened or damaged, meaning the acid flies straight into the throat because nothing prevents it from doing so anymore. The acid also irritates the surrounding tissue since your esophagus isn't built to withstand stomach acid.

The reasons why the LES muscle doesn't close are incredibly varied, as GERD can have a diet, hormonal, psychological or anatomical cause. No two people are the same. However, overwhelmingly from what I have experienced myself and what people on my YouTube channel have told me, stress and diet are the two most significant factors as to why someone develops GERD. Though, that doesn't mean these are your personal triggers.

Another issue that can cause GERD, acid reflux, or heartburn symptoms is having low or weak stomach acid. That's right. You may not have 'too much stomach acid' after all!

Many people don't know that stomach acid production can decrease with age. A poor diet, stress and nutritional deficiencies don't help the cause either. Essentially from what I can understand having done extensive research on the topic, is that you can end up eating foods that are more acidic than your stomach can handle, or there is simply a lack of stomach acid to properly digest the food. Also, stress can also affect both the quality and the quantity of your stomach acid, thus causing physical changes to your digestion.

Either way, issues with your stomach acid can cause severe pain, and you can struggle to get on top of the problem because you wrongly assume you have too much acid. The medication you'll be offered also looks to treat from the 'too much acid' angle, when really you need to address the root cause of the problem, which is *usually* diet and lifestyle related.

If GERD is left untreated, it can cause a whole host of chronic problems, which include bleeding, ulcers and internal scarring. In 10% to 15% of cases, GERD leads to Barrett's esophagus, which is when the tissue of the esophagus changes to resemble that of your intestines. This, in turn, increases your chance of developing esophageal adenocarcinoma, which is a form of stomach cancer.

Now, I know when you Google something as trivial as 'why did I sneeze?', the word cancer comes up. It's a terrifying word, and by no means will every person with GERD develop cancer, as it's thankfully very rare. But, curing your GERD is in your best interests, not least because it's impossible to function properly with it, even if you take the potential of developing cancer out of the equation. So I encourage you to make every effort here, whether you've been suffering for days or decades.

Remember, you're here researching a cure, so you're doing the right thing instead of carrying on ignoring your symptoms as others might. Please exhale now.

So what does it feel like to go through GERD? Well, whenever you say you have something 'wrong with your stomach,' people automatically assume it's something dodgy you ate that involves hours spent hurled over a toilet. But no, GERD is completely different, not least because it's higher up. It's not your intestines but your *actual* stomach. The place where food sits immediately after swallowing it.

The feeling of GERD - for me at least - was like intense heat coming from my stomach. Hence, the term 'heartburn'. Only, GERD doesn't just go away like mild bouts of heartburn. You don't feel better in the morning. It stays with you. It keeps you up at night. Personally, it felt like I had a blowtorch in my stomach that was going to burn through my flesh. I also would constantly hiccup, and it felt like I had something stuck in my throat. Ultimately, I felt very weak as I could barely eat or drink properly.

As we know, with GERD, the acid in your stomach doesn't stay where it's supposed to. The LES muscle that acts as a doorway between your stomach and esophagus is sitting wide open. You go to lay down at night, and with gravity, that acid just flies up your throat. It also does this after you eat, even when you're still upright.

The usual things that help your stomach don't work. Even

ginger feels like the equivalent of a grenade going off in there. In fact, most things make it worse. You feel weak, tired, exhausted all of the time. You aren't getting in your usual amount of nutrients or calories. When you head to the doctor, you aren't given any advice about what to eat or what not to eat. But you are given tablets that reduce your stomach acid, which actually only make the problem worse because too much acid isn't usually the problem. The problem is with the acid itself and the muscles that are supposed to be keeping that acid in. The acid can also be the wrong pH, or there simply might not be enough of it. Or, you may have an unrelated cause, such as an anatomical defect. Hence, GERD is stupidly difficult to understand as a patient, which really doesn't help when you're in the thick of it, does it?

Every time you go to a restaurant you have to be really careful what you order. Even a slice of lemon in a glass of water can make you feel instantly horrendous because lemon is acidic. People around you don't understand and might even mock you for just being 'picky' or 'difficult'. You worry about going out at all because you have to be so careful about the type of food you order. The fact that nobody understands only adds to your stress, which in turn makes your GERD worse.

So in a word, GERD is miserable. Absolutely miserable. It affected me that badly that I wrote a whole book on it in between having a jammed work schedule. I had to get my experience down for others to read because I couldn't believe just how many people were going through the same thing, equally without a clue how to get past it.

1.1 GERD SYMPTOMS

- Abdominal discomfort
- Bringing up acid into the throat
- Burning sensation in the chest
- Chest pain/tightness
- Chronic cough
- Constant hiccuping/burping
- Difficulty swallowing
- Nausea
- Poor sleep quality
- Post-nasal drip
- Sensation of a lump in the throat
- Wearing away of tooth enamel
- Worsened asthma
- Vomiting

It's good to remember that not every person will have the exact same symptoms for every medical condition, let alone GERD. As an example, I know someone who had appendicitis and had to have his appendix urgently removed. Apart from some right-sided pain, he had none of the other common symptoms.

For me, heat in my stomach, pain, loss of appetite and extreme hiccuping were my main symptoms. Air was just stuck in my throat. I want to describe it as 'difficulty swallowing' because it kind of was, only the problem was more everything I swallowed brought up horrible lumps of air too. This would happen even if eating plain foods or sipping water.

My stomach would not just rumble but full on roar super loudly. Then it would give me anxiety because everyone would hear it, and I had coworkers comment that I should go eat - yes, if only it was that simple! I have never experienced anything like it before. The thing is, I wasn't actually feeling hungry - I felt really unwell and weak and certainly didn't have an appetite. Whenever I would eat food, as soon as I swallowed anything, my stomach burned intensely, making it a miserable never-ending cycle.

In the end, I used to buy grapes and eat them at my desk because they were basically full of water, but they gave me enough sustenance to stop my stomach screaming without also giving it food that would bring the acid up. In work meetings, I would always take candy in with me to chew undetected because if it went quiet, I knew my stomach would scream.

As I said, I had no appetite. I couldn't even swallow properly. When I did eat, my stomach felt like I had poured lighter fuel into a raging fire. The burning was so sharp and long-lasting I felt like I was slowly morphing into a dragon that was about to start breathing fire. My symptoms went on for months with no sign of relief.

I also had a lot of sharp pain underneath the bottom of my left rib cage. The doctor told me that 'they only worry if it's on the right side'. But still, it was pretty uncomfortable and would make me stop whatever I was doing to breathe through it.

1.2 WHAT CAUSES GERD?

- Anxiety
- Asthma
- Being overweight
- Diet
- General eating habits
- Genetic predisposition
- Hiatal hernia
- Hormonal changes
- Magnesium deficiency
- Malfunctioning LES
- Medications
- Overeating
- Poor posture
- Pregnancy
- Smoking (including passive)
- Strenuous exercise
- Stress
- Tight fitting clothing
- Various medical conditions

The above are some of the most common GERD triggers. Some are diet related, others are to do with lifestyle, and others can even be anatomically related. There's also a very long list of medications that can trigger GERD, which frustratingly you may need to treat a different condition, but then develop GERD as a result.

For me personally, my main GERD triggers are stress, anxiety and diet. Hence, there have been occasions where I've been eating perfectly healthy, but I've had a stressful experience and my symptoms have flared up. Interestingly, a GERD friendly diet still helps to resolve my symptoms because the stress has caused a physical change in my stomach. However, I also look to address what has caused me to feel stressed or anxious in the first place. So, you may also have several different triggers too.

Because GERD is so complex, your trigger may even be something completely unrelated to the known causes, meaning yours continues to get undiagnosed. But hopefully, the above list will get your thinking cap on to try and narrow down what's making your body freak out so badly. Let's take a look at some of the main causes of GERD in greater detail.

Poor Wellbeing

So much of what we put into our bodies and what we expose ourselves to in general is a combination of being acidic, inflammatory or highly stressful. All of which keeps our bodies in a heightened state of alert making us sick from the inside out.

For example, waking up with a strong cup of coffee and a cigarette, then rushing to work on a stressful commute, only to arrive at the office and face a further series of micro-stressors throughout the day. You return home, order fast food and consume alcohol to 'destress' from the day you've just had. Rinse and repeat.

If that sounds familiar, no wonder you're feeling a little rough! Believe me, I'm not out to judge, but we have to understand that if we don't create an optimal environment for ourselves as living creatures, and if we don't approach our lifestyle in the healthiest of ways, then the simple truth is we are going to feel the effects both mentally and physically. Plus, it's impossible to perform at your best when you aren't giving your mind and body what it needs either, so this way of living is basically counterintuitive.

Alcohol, fast food and smoking are all highly acidic activities that can trigger GERD. So therein lies the problem about relying on these things to get through the day, when these very things are making us sick - especially when we do them to excess. There's a science to healing from GERD that involves the pH scale, and we'll be covering this in great detail.

But for now, think of your body as a plant. If you want it to grow big and tall and have it produce the most beautiful of blooms, you have to get the foundations right. Would shutting a plant away from sunlight, using poor quality soil and never watering it encourage it to bloom? No.

So how do you expect you - a living human being - to thrive if you're not getting what you need either? Poor gut health is probably just one of a series of problems you've been experiencing if this is the case, which is why you're going to need to address your lifestyle as a whole in order to heal from GERD, and indeed any other chronic conditions that can be attributed to poor lifestyle habits.

I genuinely think most people take better care of their cars than they do themselves. They'd never put the wrong fuel in their vehicle because they know it would break down. They also wouldn't miss a service or ignore a warning light on the dashboard. Yet, too many of us ignore our own minds and bodies that are also telling us something isn't right. We don't value ourselves enough to properly address our own needs. If that's you, then this has to stop.

Anatomical Issues

Sometimes our own actions or even a physical obstruction can cause GERD. We are going to come onto this in greater detail, but essentially if you eat then immediately lie down, exercise after a large meal or are prone to slouching, then you are fighting a losing battle against gravity. That's because your stomach contents are going to get pushed in the wrong direction.

Some people may also have a hiatal hernia that is physically restricting the normal flow of their stomach into their intestines. This, of course, is something that needs diagnosing via an upper GI endoscopy. So please ask your doctor to schedule this if they haven't already if a hernia is suspected, so you know what you're dealing with.

For those who haven't come across the term before, think of a hiatal hernia as a river that is being prevented from flowing properly due to the riverbank suddenly going uphill or even because of a massive rock in the way. That water isn't going to continue around the bend, it will get stuck or even backtrack on itself. The same thing is essentially being repeated inside your esophagus if an anatomical reason such as a hernia, is behind your GERD.

With a hernia, what's happened is the stomach has bulged through the diaphragm into the chest cavity. Since your stomach isn't sitting where it's supposed to be, neither is your food.

Your doctor may suggest a change in diet, lifestyle habits or surgery may be needed to correct the problem. Of course, if there's a chance that you can fix the problem yourself conservatively, this is always the better option, so have a thorough discussion with them.

This book is geared towards healing GERD that has a diet or lifestyle cause rather than an anatomical defect, but I do hope my tips will be useful all the same regardless of your personal cause, as these tips can help you to learn how to avoid GERD from other common triggers in the future.

Diet

I think we all know that diet lies at the heart of most illnesses and diseases. Well, GERD is no exception. Diet is an integral part of our overall health because it's how our body receives vitamins and nutrients. The problem is far too many of us don't align our diet with our actual selves. We eat the wrong foods for the wrong reasons. We self medicate with it. We indulge far too much. Therefore, you aren't going to beat GERD without taking a strong look at your diet, including not just what you eat but how you do so too.

Sadly, obesity is now a grave problem, with an estimated 1.9 billion adults now overweight across the globe, which works out as roughly one in three people. The craziest thing is that often, those who are overweight are known as 'overfed yet undernourished', i.e. the food may be giving them calories, but not the nutrients the body needs, so they continue to feel hungry. Many processed foods are also deliberately designed to contain ingredients that the brain becomes addicted to, which is why many foods are hard to kick.

Given obesity is one of the biggest causes of GERD due to the increased pressure that is placed onto the stomach, if this applies to you, then you can no longer afford to ignore your weight. I know talking about weight makes us feel uncomfortable in today's society, but speaking strictly in terms of GERD recovery, you need to give it everything you've got. Otherwise, you're severely reducing the chances of beating this thing, not to mention feeling like the best you've ever felt in your whole life.

There are some cases where GERD is completely unrelated to diet, and also, just because you have GERD it doesn't mean you're overweight. For example, I had severe GERD, and I was not overweight when I developed it. However, you may still want to use this opportunity to cut out any bad habits as you undergo your transformation since a poor diet could become a future trigger. It may also be making you feel generally sluggish in yourself without even realising it if you are heavier than you should be.

Remember - our diet is the main way our body receives nutrients, so can you say with 100% certainty that you are giving your body everything it needs to thrive and ward off chronic illness and diseases?

Also, if you suspect you may have any food allergies, then now would be a good time to get tested. Dairy, wheat and gluten can be particularly bothersome for some people. An elimination diet may be in order to narrow down anything triggering other health problems. That's not to say this will necessarily cure your GERD, but it will certainly help if your body isn't absorbing anything it can't handle or if your digestion in general always seemed to be off even before you developed GERD.

As an example, I mostly drink plant-based milk. I notice whenever I consume dairy products that use cow's milk, I immediately get inflammation in my throat, and it even makes me cough. So, we definitely need to be more aware of what we are putting in our bodies, especially in terms of chronic health conditions such as GERD.

A last point on the diet note is that you must look out for symptoms of vitamin and nutrient deficiencies on a regular basis. Of course, with GERD, you become restricted in what you can eat, which may lead to deficiencies anyway, but in general, having deficiencies in the likes of vitamin C, vitamin D/D3, vitamin B12, iron, calcium, magnesium, and zinc can throw your immune system and energy levels off.

While you should look to eat a balanced diet so that your

body can get what it needs, I also supplement with a daily multivitamin to ensure my vitamins and nutrients remain topped up. If your eating has been off for some time due to GERD, you may want to get a blood test to check your levels just to see if anything needs attention.

Mental Health

Have you ever noticed that whenever we get nervous or anxious, we feel it in our stomach? That's because the mind and the body are closely connected. The long and short of it is that if your mental health isn't in a good place, this can seriously impact your digestion. GERD is no exception.

Serotonin which is responsible for warding off depression is found in the enteric nervous system, which is located in the gut. Serotonin also affects our sleep and overall digestion, and so boosting our levels of serotonin starts with fixing not just our diet but how we look after ourselves mentally too.

In other words, a hectic lifestyle, burning the candle at both ends, surrounding yourself with toxic people and neglecting your needs ain't it.

In today's society, more of us than ever are feeling stressed, depressed, anxious or a combination of all of these. We don't know how to properly take care of our mental health, mainly because mental health has been a taboo topic for far too long.

Take GERD as the sign you've been looking for if any of this sounds familiar, since a poor mental state can create physical symptoms in the body, and GERD or, at the very least, heartburn can soon follow.

Smoking

You don't need me to tell you smoking is bad. We all know it is. We've all seen the blackened lung pictures on cigarette packets and read the cancer stats. Yet, why do so many of us still do it? So if you're a smoker and nothing up to now has made you want to quit, hopefully fixing your GERD will give you the nudge you need. Otherwise, I really don't think any other measure will be as nearly effective as it could be.

If you don't already know why smoking is bad for you, I'm not sure my words are going to make a difference. But, talking of GERD specifically, smoking is one of the worst things you can do as tobacco is a highly acidic substance.

I also want to tell you not to stand around others who are smoking because without realising it, you'll be inhaling cigarette fumes, which aside from passive smoking causing lung damage, it will most certainly trigger a flare. For me personally, the smell of smoke actually causes me to feel nauseous. As well as bringing up acid, it can put me off my food for a couple of days afterwards if it's that bad. Remember, the smell of smoke will linger on clothes and in your hair, so it can be incredibly difficult to remove from your personal environment once you've been exposed to it.

Studies have also shown that smoking decreases gastric acid secretion, which is the amount of stomach acid you need to digest food and absorb nutrients, along with gastric mucosal blood flow. Either of these issues could easily trigger your GERD symptoms.

So whether it's you who is smoking or you are around others who smoke - just don't do it. Your recovery is going to stall if you don't listen to this, regardless of how much you improve your diet or reduce your stress. This includes whether you smoke regular cigarettes or any other kind of substances - when it comes to the pH scale, the actual act of smoking or indeed vaping is, as I mentioned, highly acidic.

Your Stomach Acid Explained

Seeing as it's giving you so much grief, it might be helpful to learn what exactly your stomach acid is and what it's supposed to do. That way, when it comes to healing your GERD or even milder heartburn symptoms, you can have a better understanding of what the problem is along with the best way to treat it, or better still, avoid your symptoms in the first place!

Stomach acid is a colourless fluid that is produced by the lining of your stomach. Its purpose is to help you break down food so that your body can absorb nutrients.

Experts suggest that the normal pH of stomach acid is anywhere from 1.0 to 3.0. However, the pH of stomach acid can increase, making it less effective. This means that if you do consume anything acidic, it could well be the case that these foods are more acidic than the stomach acid designed to process the food and break it down. Or there simply might not be a big enough pH contrast between the two meaning the stomach acid is ineffective at its job.

Some people can also have a normal stomach acid pH but low levels of the stomach acid itself. Chronically low stomach acid is called hypochlorhydria, and many of the symptoms of this condition are the same as GERD.

Symptoms of hypochlorhydria include:

- Bloating
- Indigestion
- Feeling like you want to eat even when you're not hungry
- Feeling too full after regular meals
- Heartburn
- Nausea
- Soreness or burning in your mouth
- Stomach upset and cramps

Although the medication for hypochlorhydria is different to GERD, dietary changes and a reduction in stress are also recommended as a fix, so hopefully, if that's you, you'll find everything in this book just as helpful. Sadly, you may struggle to find out whether you have weak stomach acid or too little stomach acid as such tests aren't normally offered.

Instead, they give you medication to reduce stomach acid and send you on your way. Hence why so many of you are left in agony.

Another issue we've already mentioned is that the LES muscle containing your stomach acid can also be sitting loose instead of closed, meaning the acid travels upwards where it's not designed to be. As stomach acid is extremely acidic, it can cause changes in the esophagus and even erode tooth enamel if it comes into contact with either.

So if any of these things are at play, it's safe to say your food isn't going to be going down properly, and you're likely in pain or serious discomfort every time you try and swallow anything. The key is to bring the body back into balance first by letting it recover without throwing acidic foods at it that it probably can't handle, focusing on good nutrition, and reducing stress and anxiety that can affect stomach acid from a mental health perspective.

As mentioned, if your GERD is caused by a hiatal hernia or pregnancy, diet or lifestyle changes may not completely help as these are not the cause of your issue. Really, this segment and much of my book content is based on GERD, where the stomach acid is for whatever reason acting up, as this is what I experienced as a patient.

Go and get a proper diagnosis with a specialist so you know what you are dealing with if you haven't already so you can move ahead correctly with your healing strategy.

Did You Know Your Stomach Acid Levels Can Fluctuate?

Both age and even the time of the day can affect your levels of stomach acid, along with stress, zinc deficiencies, certain medications, bacterial infections or previous stomach surgery. While there are specific conditions I've mentioned above where someone can have chronically low stomach acid, in this instance, I'm talking in a general sense as part of the normal ebb and flow of the day.

A decreased amount of stomach acid can make it more difficult for you to digest your food and give off heartburn or GERD symptoms, especially if there's a misalignment with what you are eating and the amount of acid you have to digest it.

So, definitely give this some thought as you navigate eating with GERD since it's not always a level playing field. There are going to be times when you find it easier to eat versus others.

Your body is also good at letting you know when you're hungry versus when you're not. Personally, I find eating earlier in the day is better for my digestion, though everyone is going to be different.

1.3 HEARTBURN VS GERD

A common question people ask is, what's the difference between heartburn and GERD? Well, heartburn is something that most people experience at some point in their life. For example, after eating a big meal or consuming indulgent foods at Christmas. It's something that will go away on its own and typically doesn't occur very often at all.

The term 'heartburn' refers to pain felt in the centre of the chest, which is actually where the stomach sits. If we overeat or eat fatty foods, this can put pressure on the stomach, and the LES valve can open. This means your stomach acid can freely travel upwards into your esophagus or even your throat where it's not supposed to be.

Usually, you'll get that 'burny sick' feeling in the back of your throat, especially if you try to lie down. Your stomach may feel uncomfortable. But when you wake up, you'll feel fine and can eat and drink as normal.

However, GERD is when the symptoms of heartburn are both chronic and more severe. I personally had the symptoms every single day for 18 months. That means no, I didn't feel better in the morning or even a couple of months down the line. I had to be extremely careful with every single thing I ate or drank. It is all consuming because GERD is with you all the time with no letup.

If you're reading this and you get heartburn occasionally, but you don't have GERD, you will still find the tips in this book useful. In fact, I'd recommend you take note so that your heartburn doesn't develop into full-blown GERD, which I can promise you is about as fun as it sounds.

What Is Silent Reflux?

As if getting to grips with terms such as GERD, acid reflux, and heartburn wasn't enough, we also have another one to add into the mix, and that's silent reflux which is also known as laryngopharyngeal reflux (LPR).

In short, silent reflux is also a condition whereby stomach acid also flows back up through the esophagus, but it doesn't give patients the typical chest symptoms as is the case with GERD or heartburn.

Hence, people may well have symptoms and not be aware of the origin of the problem since they may notice they cough more or have a post-nasal drip, but don't realise that the issue is actually being caused by their stomach.

Symptoms Of Silent Reflux

- Asthma (the perception of)
- Chronic cough
- Hoarseness
- Noisy breathing
- Difficulty feeding in infants
- Difficulty gaining weight

The causes of silent reflux overlap with GERD. However, the symptoms present somewhat differently because they are being felt more in the throat.

Sufferers may go for years with a cough they can't get rid of, feeling as if they constantly have to clear their throat. Yet, they don't have any formal lung conditions or infections, and cough medications don't seem to help. Some people even believe they have symptoms of asthma, yet tests will prove otherwise.

Infants are also prone to silent reflux because their esophagus isn't yet fully developed, and they also spend much of their time laying down, which inhibits digestion. I have seen babies being prescribed antacids for this problem, and while I cannot give advice in place of a doctor, I do not understand why this is done, when it's clear gravity and age are at play here rather than the need to 'mop up excess acid'. But until we change perceptions about what reflux actually is, this will continue to be the way the condition is handled. It's also difficult because, naturally, parents want to reach a fast conclusion to ease the symptoms their child is experiencing. I hope more research will be conducted in this area by the medical world.

The good news is that for adults, healing from silent reflux follows much of the same advice that is given to GERD patients. So, I'm hoping you, too, will find relief if you happen to be suffering from silent reflux as opposed to GERD. At the very least, you'll know what it is now!

1.4 MY GERD STORY

Imagine you've just started a new job. You had to guess your start date due to extremely vague communication from your boss. When you arrive on your first day, the colleague you're supposed to shadow is in hospital with appendicitis, so they don't know what to do with you. There's no computer for you to be able to start your official duties. You have no qualifications that match anyone else on your team as you were brought into the company as part of a brand new role. The office is so tense you can hear a pin drop because the office also happens to be a newsroom, and you've walked straight into them covering a horrific case involving the concealment of a dead baby. This is week one.

Your inability to assist your team does not go unnoticed by the receptionist, who insists you make yourself useful by 'dealing' with an angry woman in reception, who has arrived suitcase in tow in case she is sent to prison that day. She is unhappy that her criminal case has been made public, and she wants you to 'sort it'. You have no idea who she is, what she has been charged for or indeed what she could potentially do to you, given there isn't security at reception, let alone a metal detector.

Your job is supposed to be working *behind the scenes*, writing up content for a news website. You are now casually wondering to yourself if you're about to get stabbed.

No, I haven't momentarily slipped into fiction writing. This was indeed the real introduction I had to a job that led to such acute stress and burnout I developed GERD as a result. I lost the ability to eat and drink properly and indeed function due to the experience.

As we've covered, stress is something that can have serious implications for our health. Given work is where most of us spend the majority of our time, and it is what we rely on to generate an income to survive, it's little wonder that our employment can be a trigger for any number of health conditions. This is especially the case when employees are overworked and undervalued, and there's a toxic management culture, in conjunction with daily abuse from the public just for doing your job, as was the case for me.

Such workplaces make it impossible for their employees to thrive at their jobs by setting unrealistic standards. In fact, all they do is create a culture of misery, and ultimately, their employees and, therefore, the company will never reach its potential. Neither will you as an individual as long as you stay. If you're like me, not being able to give the job your all because of the conditions of the job itself will be one of the most deeply frustrating aspects of the whole debacle.

A job I had applied to with great enthusiasm, I might add, as the publication had always been a staple in our house growing up. As a child, I used to scrape together the money to purchase a copy out of the coins my eldest eldest brother had scattered along our hallway after returning from a night out. I remember counting out the 27 pence exactly, which is what a copy of the publication cost back then. My work had also been published in it as far back as when they used to print a junior edition some decades ago.

It's worth noting that this newsroom no longer exists, and the publication has changed its name from when I first started. My story is not about identifying the publication or anyone involved, rather highlighting what a complete disregard for employee wellbeing can result in for ***any company*** and indeed its employees. It's so often something that nobody dares to talk about, let alone address, meaning such behaviours remain unchecked. This leaves things wide open for the next unsuspecting person to join the company repeating the cycle and thus the misery all over again.

I'm sure you're all familiar with newspapers and online news websites, though you probably don't appreciate just how much content is needed every single day - it's a 24/7 operation. Often, a very small team is responsible for sourcing the stories, writing them up, getting them published on the website, monitoring social media inboxes, answering calls and emails about incoming stories, plus dealing with public feedback from the ones that have already been printed. Sometimes on weekends or holidays, it can literally be one person sitting alone in an office responsible for all of that, including someone like me, who doesn't even have any journalism qualifications.

All this is against the backdrop of woefully low salaries with 12 hours a week unpaid overtime written into your contract. The CEO, of course, receives record-breaking bonuses and eye-watering amounts of company shares each year while denying even the most minuscule of wage increases for the workforce that have generated that revenue. But, they are happy to announce plenty of redundancies. This is far from a unique story, I'm sure.

I knew something was off during the interview stage when I was asked "how would you cope if we sent you to a murder scene?" and asked to justify why I didn't know shorthand, when the role was not to be a journalist but to work within digital content. Yes, the job was to work within a newsroom, but my role would be to support the fast rotation of written content on the website, rather than to actively go out in the field because, you know, I am not a journalist, nor have I applied to be one.

I was also asked whether "this is just a job you'll do for six months before you quit." Not exactly standard questions you prepare answers for when you have a job interview. I'd literally come prepared to talk about their SEO strategy.

When a colleague who sat in on the interview called to offer me the job a few weeks later, I thought they had made a mistake because I felt woefully unprepared for every question I had been asked and frankly way out of my depth. I decided to go against my intuition and accept the job.

This was my first ever job where I was being hired as an actual writer aside from on freelance platforms. I was the only person to be working on the newsroom team with no formal qualifications in the field, and in short, it was quite the gig to have landed based on these facts. So, you can only imagine how badly I wanted it to work out, and in hindsight, maybe this clouded my judgement with what I was prepared to put up as time went on.

The colleague I was supposed to shadow returned from having his appendix removed a couple of weeks after I started. He'd heard it through the grapevine that I hadn't been settled into the job properly yet. He told me how he'd returned early as he didn't want me to quit on them, especially since I was hired to reduce his impossible workload, which saw him working many hours over his quota each day. I was relieved he was so nice because up to now, I had just felt like I was in the way of everyone else.

Fast forward to a few weeks in the job, and this same colleague takes his annual leave as I'm now there to cover some of his workload. But I think fine, he's shown me the ropes, so I know what I need to do.

Out of the blue, an email arrived from my boss, stating my performance so far was 'disappointing' and that he was on his way in to see me. I wracked my brain to try and think what on earth he could be referring to since I had only been in the job for less than a month at this point and couldn't for the life of me work out what I'd supposedly done wrong. I was sitting working on the tasks my colleague had told me I needed to concentrate on, crossing them off in my notepad one by one.

So I decided to ask my line manager to get a second opinion. Now, this wasn't to double-cross my boss, rather to try and ascertain any major issue that had yet to be brought to my attention because they had daily meetings together, and as I mentioned, I was genuinely at a loss here. I had tried to keep out of the way of all the tension in the newsroom and not cause an issue for anyone. I was just trying to get on with my job behind the scenes of what we did as a publication.

I said to my line manager that firstly, I was working on 'XYZ', and if this isn't correct, then please let me know so I can give you what you need from me. She told me not to worry because my performance was absolutely fine and that my boss was simply struggling in his quest to go vegan. That was it. That was the chat.

About half an hour later, my boss comes in and summons me to his office to demand why I hadn't replied to his email. I said to him that I thought the tone was off, considering he hadn't been specific about what he wanted and that I'd discussed it with my line manager to see if there was anything else they needed from me other than the work I was doing to cover my colleague, and she said no.

Also, as a content writer, tone in digital communication is exceptionally important. So to write an extremely stern email to a new person in the job is really, really strange, especially as they knew my start hadn't gone to plan and this wasn't my fault. Needless to say, I felt overwhelmed with worry.

The big issue? He didn't like the way I had scheduled tweets on Twitter, as I had made a few repeats to pad the timeline out. Something you know you can instantly delete if you're not happy with. Or better still, outline how you would like the Twitter feed to be run for your company before insisting your newest member of staff take the reins so that you don't create even the slightest possibility they could mess it up for you. Believe it or not, I would never have wanted to mess it up for them either.

The experience rattled me so much I started to feel very anxious. That's because it felt like this was an authority asserting exercise so that I knew my place, rather than me having actually done anything 'wrong', especially not to warrant that level of a telling off. As you may know, when you feel anxious it actually has an impact on your appetite and digestive system. For me this initially appeared as a weird pain and a lack of appetite. I'd never really experienced this before, so I figured it would go away on its own.

But it didn't. I felt unable to switch off from work due to these constant interactions where I was being pulled up for things that I couldn't have possibly known. So the next time I was called in the office, I interjected that they needed to outline any future things so that they were being fair, which at that stage they clearly were not. Because up to now, it felt like they had been laying traps since I explicitly asked everyone around me if they needed anything. Yet there would always be *something* new to find fault with, no matter what I did. Only instead of recognising this as me taking initiative, it only seemed to make my boss get even more frustrated with me because he seemed to interpret this as highlighting his failures when he was determined to keep the focus on mine as a warped form of stress release. I just couldn't win.

So I tried to look for other opportunities to show I was committed to the job. Management were very precious about posting stories on Facebook in particular because it would immediately create a traffic surge for the website. They needed as many website views as possible because of the advertising revenue it would bring. Before I left in the evenings, I would often be responsible for scheduling all the Facebook posts and tweets, or if working weekends it would be my sole responsibility to look after socials.

I noticed my line manager was really bogged down in a case and very stressed. It had been a few hours since a post had gone out. I knew that we were due a post, but everyone was too busy to do it. I didn't want to add to their stress by having the socials slip when these were so crucial to page views and revenue. So I asked a colleague next to me whether I should post on the Facebook page to help my line manager out, and she thought it was a good idea.

I took one of our newer stories that hadn't appeared on the feed that day, created an appropriate message for it and sent it out. The post did alright, and website traffic started to flood in on our giant analytics monitor screen.

Within five minutes, my line manager appears from over her computer screen and goes ballistic at me in an expletive laden rant. A deathly silence immediately cut across the entire office. She mumbles something about having a very specific format for Facebook and that it's 'not my job' to decide what goes out and when.

Now, although my boss was more acidic in nature than any GERD triggering food, my line manager wasn't a horrible person. I actually recognised this person was overloaded with stress, so I tried to not take it personally. However, a few weeks later they then swore at me again, telling me to "eat your fucking sweet", after a misunderstanding that I couldn't respond to them at that precise second because I was eating. I was literally just swallowing something, so I meant it as an awkward joke - I was mortified it came off as anything but.

Add to this some of the case details you'd hear as part of your average day, as I mentioned, and it certainly didn't help my mental health. Now, I'm not naive. I appreciate working in journalism means you will be exposed to the best and worst of humanity with severe emphasis on the worst. It's also your duty to bring the information to the people and I was fully aware of this responsibility. But I noticed there seemed to be no discussion on how to not absorb details of what you were working on. Or how to deal with people screaming at you down the phone. It was either you're tough, and you don't get fazed by it, or you're not, and if you're not, don't expect to find any support.

The more I internalised everything, the more my body would react, and this then impacted my appetite. I noticed that when I swallowed food, my stomach would be really painful. I started to get worried, so I went to the doctor, and he initially prescribed me some tablets that relax your stomach before you eat. I also tried over the counter tablets for anxiety to see if it would help me feel calmer at work. I thought this would be enough to solve my symptoms since I had never experienced any major digestive issues before.

One day, I arrived extra early to work as I knew my colleague would be off, and I wanted to get a headstart on the day. It got to 1.30 pm, and I had worked solidly without a break due to how busy the newsroom was since about 8am. My boss had asked me to do a task, which I had started. I saw everyone else leave for lunch, including him, and I figured since I had been there for more than five hours already without a break, it would be okay if I took my half an hour lunch break too. I knew I needed to take my medication and have a quick bite to eat with it as prescribed.

I was gone for all of 20 minutes, and when I returned, my boss was extremely cross and called me into his office yet again, demanding to know where I had been. I explained I had been there since before everyone else had got in and that I needed to take my medication for my stomach. Since I'd passed the legal limit for how long you can work without a break, I thought surely this isn't going to be a problem, especially as I was as quick as I could be - not even using my full supposed 'lunch break' of 30 minutes. He simply replied that I had "had a shaky start to this job" and ordered me to go home until I felt better. His tone of voice was most certainly not of concern, I can tell you that much. I had failed him, yet again. Just for taking a lunch break and not even all of it either.

We're only a month or so into the job, and I return having had a couple of days off from being sent home. I was made to complete a 'return to work' interview, which is basically a way of shaming you for being ill. No, my stomach didn't feel better, and yes, I was full of anxiety. But what the hell can you do when you've only just started in a job, and this is how it's going so far?

I was also told how it had been noted that I was leaving on time in the evening and that this was deeply frowned upon. From now on, I needed to go around asking people if they needed anything before I was allowed to leave at night. Realising I was now being monitored when I took a break or indeed left for work, I never left work on time from that point onwards. Even though I had genuinely finished all of my tasks, and despite the fact I was always one of the first people in, meaning I was already giving them more time than they realised.

I went back to my doctor at this point because I felt extremely anxious about my work situation, and it was affecting my eating more than ever. The diagnosis then moved onto gastritis which is an inflammation of the stomach lining. The only advice he gave me was "not to eat crisps." I now didn't dare leave my seat for any amount of noticeable time in case I got in trouble again with my boss, so I'd turned to such junk convenience food.

When I did take a break, I had to make sure I had scheduled

enough tweets to cover my absence - yes, even if I was gone for a few minutes. We would usually eat lunch at our desk because you only got a short half-hour break, which isn't as long as it sounds when you're working in an incredibly tense atmosphere. It was also difficult to take a break because, with news, it's impossible to switch off. If something happens, you need to be on it immediately.

A big story would come in, and the tone would change, sandwiches would be dropped, and you'd need to muck in and write something or check social media for additional information. From a news perspective, I absolutely get this. However, the problem is that the reality of being ready to spring to action at all times doesn't compute with how we as humans work, especially when you are in a perpetual state of high alert. It means that even when you leave work at night, you can never truly switch off in case you miss something.

Also, it was clear that the newsroom had a back to front workweek. On a Monday, the atmosphere would be fairly relaxed unless any big stories came in. But towards the end of the week, when you naturally start to tire, you'd actually have to pick up the pace several gears because you'd need to prepare content for Saturday and Monday's edition in the same amount of time because they didn't have weekend or night time staff like larger newsrooms - we had to do it all. A Friday afternoon was the tensest time of all, and I once witnessed someone weep at their desk when it all got too much. The more I experienced in the job, the more I absorbed, and the worse my stomach pain got.

How most people would cope with the stress of the job was to smoke - a lot. I have never smoked, but I have always had an issue with people smoking near me because the smell of stale smoke makes me feel sick, due to me having particularly potent smell aversions. So imagine how I felt when so many people around me were constantly running off to smoke then sitting back down near me. I get they had to do it to relieve the pressure of the job, but I constantly felt nauseous because of it. This really didn't help the burning pain in my stomach and the acid that was now coming up into my throat because of the constant stress and anxiety I felt, coupled with the putrid smell of cigarettes.

As part of my job, I also had to do food reviews of local restaurants. Now, normally that would have been a dream, but because so many foods were causing burning pain and acid in my throat, I would dread it. I even asked to be taken off the list of food reviewers. To them, I'm sure it sounded like I wasn't committed to the job, but I was genuinely at my wits' end with the feeling of burning in my stomach and chest. I could barely eat my own food, let alone anyone else's.

I'd do it anyway because the food review had a slot to fill in the publication. Otherwise, they would be short on content, and this would create even more stress for everyone. So, I'd try and order the plainest thing on the menu, but usually, it would still feel like I had swallowed molten lava. There was one time I ate a lasagne, and it took about a week for the pain in my stomach to subside because of the layers of oozing fatty cheese that sat on top of it.

At this point, I was drinking ginger tea to 'settle my stomach', as ginger especially is good for stomach pain under normal circumstances. Only, this is not the case for GERD (which I didn't know I had yet) because it only intensifies the heat as you swallow. Of course, it only made things worse.

Having returned to my doctor yet again, he put me on omeprazole. I also was told to take 'the pink goo', which is my description of liquid antacid medication. This was my doctor's suggestion to make the burning feeling go away, with no real explanation of what acid reflux or GERD actually is. I wasn't even told that omeprazole is given for acid reflux, GERD or heartburn. So, I was still very much in the dark about what was actually wrong with me and how to help myself, other than taking these two medications. This also meant I wasn't researching GERD specific diets or healing strategies, because the information wasn't being relayed. Only the medication to treat it.

I made a valiant effort to take everything as prescribed. I will say 'the pink goo' did help settle the acid after I tried to eat. The problem was the effect was only very temporary. All of my symptoms would come back. I was also drinking about ten cups of camomile tea a day just to settle my stress at work. But, I still wasn't getting to the root of what was actually up with me, let alone how to fix it.

In an office filled to the brim with lots of people, it could work one of several ways. On a Friday evening - our most stressful point of the week - the advertising department down the far end of the room would find it courteous to hold a big, loud party. You'd be desperately trying to concentrate on getting the weekend stuff written up to the deadline, while grown adults blasted out 'Conga' by Black Lace in the background. You wondered whether a rolled up copy of our publication thrown at speed would be worth the disciplinary action for the five minutes' peace it would give you.

Other times, there would be a deafening silence especially when a big story was in process.

However, the worst was when my boss would walk in around 10.30am and the mood would instantly change. The casual chit chat you had with your colleagues that dampened down your imposter syndrome for those precious few minutes would immediately cease. I noticed this is when my symptoms really ramped up. My whole body would go rigid with the tension. Because I knew the word 'Rachael!' was coming, along with an order or a critique after it.

The crazy thing was, despite me constantly being pulled up for the most random of things, in my job itself, I was bringing in some big stories for the team. Not that anyone would ever acknowledge this, of course.

For one of the stories I found, I came across a social media post saying 'RIP' under the profile picture of a company that has been in town for hundreds of years, as it had gone out of business. This was the first big scoop I made for the publication and one which turned out to be a huge rolling story. I thought finally, I've done something right, and things will surely turn a corner with my boss now. But no, that alone is not enough to impress him.

Bearing in mind my job is supposed to be in digital content as a non-journalist, my boss tells me I am to head down to the scene and interview people on video reacting to the story and that I wasn't to come back to the office until I'd done so.

I was given a notepad and paper, despite not knowing shorthand or having any journalism qualifications to know how to interview people. They knew this, and I'm fairly sure this was to humiliate me. Even a qualified journalist who started on the same day told me she panicked because she did not study broadcast journalism when given a similar task. Yet, here I was, with no journalism qualifications at all, being asked to deliver the same. Let me make it clear that I was happy to do what was needed to support my team, but I was concerned that I was not equipped with the skills to deliver what was needed to the required standard, since this fell way out of my remit as a content writer.

My YouTube channel consisted of basic beauty reviews, so yes, I knew how to capture video but not how to go up to random people and conduct an interview. Those are two *very different things*. As an introvert, there's also a reason I look to work in jobs behind the scenes. Yet you know how it is; some people recognise this as a 'weakness' in you, and decide it's their mission to 'fix' you. As if wanting to quietly get on with your work instead of being the loudest in the room is some kind of disease.

We had never discussed me having to interview the public on video before I was told to leave immediately and go do it. So instead of me embracing the challenge naturally as I grew into my role or even being able to express it wasn't something I was comfortable with, it was basically a case of go do it now, and by the way, the future existence of your role relies on what you come up with. To randomly have that placed on your shoulders in the middle of a workday is really unnerving. Then, of course, when you get back, you still have all your other work to do as a content writer, which is also time-sensitive. So now it's a combination of nerves and stress rolled into one.

Nobody would speak on camera, so terrified I was going to lose my job if I 'messed up again' with my boss, my mum, who was a lifelong customer of the store, agreed to pose as a random member of the public. She did a brilliant job, but I can't help thinking about what would have happened if she hadn't stepped in. I also realised that despite my role not being a journalist, I was basically there to be a journalist. Alongside all my other roles such as finding stories, managing the newsroom by myself on weekends, answering the phone when nobody else would, dealing with angry members of the public, oh and writing six stories a day for the website. Got it.

Long story short, I didn't fail, and we got several ongoing stories off the one tip-off I found, though I knew I'd gone far beyond the job scope to achieve it. This was to be the standard I now had to follow, which was far more than the job description entailed. The official term for this is 'out of scope', and ironically, on the freelancing platform I now work for, it's illegal, as is unpaid overtime, which, as I mentioned, this job also required in abundance.

I kept looking out for similar story tip-offs or ideas for the online content. These successes kept coming even when I was met with impossible demands, like doing things I wasn't qualified for and weren't within my job scope. But the picture that was being painted about my ability kept on being tarnished, with constant verbal ridicules about my ability and even one occasion where my salary was read out aloud by my boss. He also once announced to the entire office that my spelling was horrendous. All little things designed to ebb away at my confidence and prove that no, you couldn't come into this world as a non-journalist and succeed. Even though I kept proving them wrong with the stories I was finding.

By this point, I was getting really sick and feeling very weak as my stomach symptoms were not settling down. I was surviving on a diet of porridge in the morning and chicken, kale, mashed potato and gravy for dinner. Sometimes I'd eat a sandwich at lunch, but then because I ate while at work, the stress would make my stomach severely burn afterwards.

I visited California over the holidays, though the job stress was so great that it never really left me. Also, when GERD starts, there is no magic tap to turn it off. So you may be away from the stress temporarily, but your stomach is still a raging fire because, in the end, the fix requires huge changes and a determined effort. But when you're on medication to reduce your stomach acid, and nobody has explained what that really means or what you should do to get better other than taking omeprazole and antacids, you continue to struggle.

Although most of the trip had been a washout due to my uncontrolled GERD symptoms (not that I fully understood this at the time), one of the places I had managed to visit in LA was Universal Studios. I decided to buy some American candy to bring back for the office because I figured it might be a way to connect with my colleagues better and hopefully put the last year behind us. I had gotten on well with most of the office, but things were still dire with my boss.

After sending out a group email telling people I brought some candy back, I noticed my boss approach the desk where I left the candy, and I thought that we might just have an ice breaker here. He took one bite and proceeded to announce to everyone that my candy "tasted like baby sick."

I felt so embarrassed that I cleared the candy away from the table and ate most of it myself to get rid of it. Unaware, of course, that chocolate is also bad for GERD because, at this point, I didn't properly understand the condition. I had a drawer full of chocolate at my desk which I would use to stress eat after each bad interaction with my boss since trying to talk to him about our differences clearly didn't work. There was no other way I was able to cope.

From this point on, the sound of him saying my name, which preceded yet another order, was a constant repetition throughout the day. No, these were not normal things your boss asks you to do. I felt like his puppet, especially when the phone would ring and I'd have to hold up the phone until he'd finished his conversation because the cable wouldn't reach and he wouldn't get up himself.

One time nobody could get into the office because of deep snowfall blocking the roads. I took public transport (something I was frequently mocked for) and actually got there before anyone else. My boss eventually makes it in around lunchtime, orders a coffee for my colleague for 'getting in early and keeping things going'. He then proceeds to quiz me at what time I arrived, assuming I'd used the weather as an opportunity to turn up late, when I was the first person in several hours ago, yes before the guy he just bought a coffee for as a thank you. I was slowly going insane, and because it was only directed at me, nobody could see it either.

Two key journalists from our very small team had also quit, and they weren't replaced for several months, meaning we were now woefully understaffed. This meant I had to take on more and more work to help maintain the flow of content, including taking on more roles where I would formally interview people or head to the scene of incidents. Despite my role being behind the scenes, it now felt like I was very much centre stage, without any of the attributes or training everyone else had while being expected to produce content to the same standard. If you don't come up with the goods, you're going to raise the levels of stress even further because of the fast turnover of content required, so you have to do it.

Answering a phone in a newsroom also is essentially a game of Russian roulette. Is it going to be an old lady who hasn't had her copy of the publication delivered, or is it someone ringing up to say their sister has been crushed to death in an industrial accident, and you're the only person available to write the story? Or, is it going to be someone threatening to physically harm you because they don't like the fact their criminal case has been made public?

All of the above happened to me, the latter on my first weekend shift when I was working alone in the office.

What most people don't realise about newsrooms is often they are the first port of call for a whole wrath of emotions, which are often incredibly raw, especially after an accident or a high profile story. When it comes to anger and particularly grief, such phone calls can be absolutely draining to deal with. Sometimes colleagues' voices would be raised, or tears would be shed, and yet others were able to keep a completely calm tone throughout.

The abusive phone calls, in particular, did not help the symptoms I was experiencing with my stomach. In fact, the pain, heat, difficulty swallowing and grinding my teeth in my sleep continued to get worse, the more I answered that phone and the more I was constantly pulled up by my boss.

But who do you tell you are struggling mentally and physically in a job? Your line manager who basically works seven days a week and is incredibly stressed with insane demands paired against a lack of staff, or your boss who is actively searching for another opportunity to reprimand you?

Then there were the painfully entitled people who it felt were put on this earth just to shave some additional stress over your impossible workload, just to enhance the taste of despair in case it wasn't quite astringent enough.

Somewhere deeply embedded in a crevice of hell, it had been cast upon me that I would be assigned to the task of managing all stories relating to a local beauty pageant. If you're assuming syrupy sweet smiles and Shirley Temple-sque poses are as ferocious as it gets, you haven't met their mothers.

You know those ridiculous hostage movies where they demand $1,000,000 in cash, a helicopter on the roof and a pizza delivered to them within the hour? The phone rings. I had a mother of a pageant entrant on the line who bluntly insisted her daughter's bake sale needed a front page tomorrow. Otherwise, she wouldn't win the publicity round of the contest, and it would be my fault if she didn't go on to win the entire thing because they really needed the points from that round to clinch the contest.

For anyone who has never submitted a story to a newspaper before, directing those who put the newspaper together where your story should rank isn't exactly how it works. Especially when one doesn't even have the seniority to suggest that, let alone implement it for you.

Instead, front pages have a commercial framework behind

them, seen as they will be the first thing people see, and will determine whether people buy that newspaper or not. So even if the entire newsroom was eaten alive by the lions and I was left as acting editor - which isn't as implausible as you might think given my town once had some animals escape from a visiting circus - your bake sale still wouldn't be getting a front page. Unless there is some other element to the story that suddenly makes it more newsworthy from a commercial standpoint. It's not me be being mean, anti-women or indeed anti-pageant not to have given her the request, it's just how publications work. You lead from the top and work your way down.

So, I placed details of this delightful sounding bake sale in the public event announcement equivalent of 'nibs' which is short for news in brief. The mother called me back a few days later and went absolutely crazy at me because I was now responsible for her daughter "not becoming famous."

Many other similar interactions with the public occurred where demands would be made to turn up at events that were not deemed newsworthy enough to take the limited staff off we had, especially when they were busy covering accidents or high profile court cases. All of these interactions took up more of your time and energy that was badly needed elsewhere, and you were always to blame because you were on the other end of the phone.

As news stories are also published on social media, and there's a comment section under articles, you'd also need to monitor what people were saying, especially if it could be libellous or expose details of a case that could put someone in danger. This was extremely important to keep an eye on, but it wasn't always easy with so much plate spinning going on at the same time.

People would also start rows over social media posts which could get particularly nasty. Then they'd call us in the newsroom for us to 'sort it out'. So you'd have to stop whatever you were doing, which was usually working to a very tight deadline to get a story up, just to stop Susan and Janice knocking seven bells out of each other on your Facebook comments.

I'd endeavour to stay professional, but sometimes the lack of logic in place of entitlement got to me. One example that springs to mind is when a lady rang up because she'd done some work in the community, and we hadn't turned up to photograph her and put her in the paper. Because you know, getting in the paper is the point of doing good work an' all. She went on and on about how we kept missing these events she was putting on. So I asked her whether she'd explicitly told us these events were happening and that we'd agreed it was newsworthy enough to send someone down. The lady replied, "I posted it on my Facebook page, you should have seen it on there." She was deeply offended that we didn't actively read every single Facebook page on the internet as part of our day. Again, this was my fault.

With the stress coming in from every angle of the job, my mental and physical symptoms were continuing to deteriorate. As I said, my doctor had prescribed omeprazole, but it only made me feel worse, never better, because the approach was to try to treat the symptom rather than the root cause as it always is with the pharmaceutical industry.

There was one day I left work on Friday and didn't eat anything until Monday because my stomach burned so badly whenever I tried to swallow anything. It had gotten to Saturday, and I really didn't feel well at all, so I called up for an out of hours appointment at my hospital. I told the nurse on the phone the omeprazole was making me feel worse, that it was just not helping, and that I felt really unwell.

So I get in there, and I see the doctor. The first comment he makes is about my handbag, stating that a 'designer' handbag was not normally seen in a hospital environment. It was the only bag I had which I could fit my medication in. It was a plain, £20 bag I had bought from Zara. Absolutely nothing designer about it. I wonder, would a man's consultation about severe abnormal pain, burning, hiccups and trouble swallowing and extreme stress and anxiety have started the same way, or am I being paranoid here?

He finally got off the topic of my dress sense and looked at my medical history. His first question was why I was bothering him when I have one of the best GPs in the area. Even though it was a Saturday, and my doctors wouldn't be open until Monday. I told him my symptoms and that I was struggling to eat. He suggested I may have an H. pylori infection, which is similar to GERD, but it still wasn't the correct diagnosis as the test came back negative. Yes, this is after I had already been prescribed omeprazole which is given to patients with GERD. Nobody was explaining the condition to me - not even doctors who could see my medical history and past prescriptions in front of them.

I left his office and started to walk out of the building when the same doctor started following me. He stops me, and announces to the entire hospital waiting room, "just to let you know, young lady, you aren't doing yourself any favours by not eating and drinking." As if I was deliberately abstaining from food when I physically couldn't swallow because every time I did, the searing heat made me want to cry, and that the medication I had been prescribed - omeprazole - only made my stomach feel drier and hotter each time I took it. As we now know, omeprazole helps to reduce the amount of acid your stomach makes when most people have **low levels of stomach acid** when they experience GERD symptoms. But no, it was me refusing to eat, which was the real reason behind my illness.

During the consultation, one thing this doctor mentioned to me was that I should drink peppermint tea as it's good for stomach problems. I was so desperate I drank several cups of it because this was the first piece of dietary advice I received from any doctor up to now. It was only later I found out peppermint tea is one of the worst things you can drink with GERD.

The peppermint moved so violently through my system it caused a part of my digestive tract to burst, resulting in me filling a toilet with about half a pint of blood. At this point, feeling so ill, burning pain in my stomach, unable to eat, crippled with stress and now having lost blood, I was extremely scared.

I returned to my GP on the following Monday. I had to have an immediate investigation because now my symptoms were overlapping with cancer. Thankfully it wasn't. But you can imagine what the experience did to my mental state, which was already in tatters by this point. Ironically, when they were doing further tests, to distract me, they asked about my job because, as I said, it's one of those publications that everyone reads. The irony.

Just to make sure the bleeding was nothing sinister, they ordered an urgent ultrasound of my abdomen. I wish I was making this up, but the sonographer had to repeat the test four times because he told me he wasn't sure what he was looking at on the screen. I'm in a hospital, and they are trying to fully rule out cancer or another urgent problem, and he doesn't know what he's looking at?

So I get back to work after my scan. I sat down and my phone rang. The head of the department was on the line, instructing me to return to the hospital so she could double check the scan herself because they weren't confident the guy had done it correctly even after the second time. After repeating the scan, she reassured me everything looked fine. I thanked her because she was a lot more professional, but I honestly thought to myself, what type of a show are you running here?

In the same hospital, I had an x-ray a few months prior, and they came out to ask me what the body part was because they had never heard of it before (a cervical rib). This level of incompetence is the very last thing you need when you are sick and worried out of your mind wondering what the hell is wrong with you, let me tell you.

I returned to my GP, who got me a referral with a gastroenterologist. At this point, my symptoms were anxiety, burning pain in my stomach, hiccuping, trouble swallowing, lack of appetite, sharp pain under my left rib and of course, the bleeding episode. It's a weird thing to say I was 'looking forward' to meeting with the gastroenterologist because that's not quite how I'd describe it. But, I was hoping he'd be able to point me in the right direction, at least as a professional in his field.

Only, the appointments we had didn't go like that. I would ask questions about why I'm having these symptoms and, crucially - what I can do to help myself. Apart from telling me I was clearly stressed and to take probiotics (which, yes, is important to know and I'm grateful), he couldn't advise me further. He said I was too young to have a camera down my throat, and surgically, there was nothing he could do for me, so he was discharging me. Yet again, no diet plan or healing strategy was mentioned. All he could tell me was that "I wasn't sixteen anymore" in relation to why my stomach was giving me such strange sensations.

The average salary for his position and seniority is £96,000 ($129,600) a year. He specialises in disorders of the digestive system and couldn't give me any advice about how to manage my GERD symptoms, when my GP had referred me to him specifically for that purpose. Just let that sink in.

I had been warned by a previous physiotherapist who had worked in hospitals for most of his career to "watch out for egotistical surgeons." He explained to me that *some surgeons* only care if they can immediately operate and get that 'macho buzz' from saving the day. If not, they genuinely don't care and just want rid of you. I thought surely that's not how it is? I'm afraid in this instance, that story I had been told was all I could think of.

Sometimes you just can't believe something until you actually experience it, and to be honest, seeing a specialist in a field who doesn't even tell you the basics such as a diet plan, how to eat with GERD, what to avoid etc., is beyond a joke, especially when their patient is specifically asking them for this information, and they are basically answering you with the same fragrant vagueness of that of a politician.

To be feeling so fragile and desperate for help, only to feel like you are constantly hitting a brick wall with every professional you encounter, is something I wouldn't wish on anyone. I wasn't trying to play the system, skip work or waste time. I just wanted a diagnosis and a treatment plan so I could go away and kick this thing because I'd had enough.

There is, in my opinion, a deep level of misogyny within the healthcare world, but that is for another book. Given how weak I felt at the time, it honestly makes me furious.

So instead, I was left to figure it out on my own. If I returned to my GP, there wouldn't be a lot else they could do because they'd already referred me to the top. It had felt like a massive waste of time, and I certainly wasn't getting any better.

All the while, I was still trying to battle through my job, and things with my boss didn't improve, which only exacerbated my symptoms.

He would make spelling mistakes in my work and change place names in the title, so I would look stupid when the content was published online. I remember getting trolled on social media for mistakes in my work I didn't even make. People (including previous employees of the publication) were contacting me to tell me I should be sacked. This is the very tip of the iceberg for online abuse anyone who works in journalism gets, meaning many are too scared to have social media profiles in their own name. Despite the fact you need a profile in your own name to

be able to contact your sources. Yes, even 'supposed-behind-the-scenes
-workers-who-didn't-apply-to-be-a-journalist-but-basically-had-to-become-one-overnight.'

Online abuse is only part of the challenge for journalists' mental health, especially when you consider journalists who are sent to war zones or disasters that may well experience serious mental trauma. The profession itself can also be incredibly dangerous. Every year, journalists are killed on the job and not just in war zones but in countries around the world, including the ones you think of as 'safe'.

All when that individual is simply trying to do their job. Hence, constant abuse from the public certainly does little to settle the feeling of unease in the profession.

Of course, stress and burnout also wear you down mentally and physically, even if you're in the confines of an office feeling completely overworked. The less you have to give, the more likely you are to snap, especially if you can't remember the last time you had a good night's sleep, oh, and you currently can't eat or drink properly due to uncontrolled GERD.

It had reached the point where the high level of unpaid overtime was really starting to exhaust me, especially one week that required me to work seven days straight due to a combination of a training course and staff shortages. The problem with unpaid overtime is that it immediately makes you less valuable because you are working for free. Only, you're not volunteering for a charity, you are making that business money. Not that those at the bottom will ever see that cash.

Burnout fast approaches. But I ploughed on. One day, I was monitoring the social media inbox, and a message came through. Someone had noticed a raid was underway at an animal rescue centre. Now, the initial message definitely played down the situation, and to be honest, we were only used to drug raids which weren't necessarily huge stories because they are a common occurrence. But, I thought it was worth investigating, so I grabbed hold of one of my colleagues who was having a chat with a photographer. I scrawled an address down and handed it to them, practically pushing them out of the door telling them to get there quickly.

The story ended up getting the publication the equivalent of a month's worth of page views in a single day - I'm talking page views in the millions. We actually broke the analytics monitor because we had that many people on our site at one time. While of course the success of the story was down to the incredible drone work from our photographer that showed the scale of the operation, and the work of the journalist I practically catapulted out of the door - if I hadn't used my intuition, we wouldn't have scooped that story. I also wrote several stories about the case that then undercovered a network of animal abuse the owner of the facility had been involved in.

Unbelievably, we had abusive phone calls about printing that story. One woman rang me up to tell me her husband was "a very wealthy man" and that he would be taking us to court because the story was all lies when we'd seen the abhorrent unpixelated versions of the conditions these animals were kept in. I don't know whether some people have an illness that makes them think they can convince others that things aren't real when there is an abundance of proof, but I could feel the tendons bulging out of her neck due to the strain in her voice. Literally, screaming at me for bringing this story to light, as if we were the ones in the wrong and not her associates who ironically, went on to be convicted of their crimes in court by a judge and jury, by the way.

A few weeks later, we all had to have individual meetings with our line manager and the boss as our roles would be changing to take on areas of special interest. Mine was helping people locally who were struggling financially, having been raised by a single parent in challenging economic circumstances myself.

My meeting (held 90 minutes after I should have clocked off, of course) went like so. Firstly, my boss claimed he didn't know I had anything to do with finding the story of the year I just mentioned. I was then shown a bar chart of the expected page views each colleague was expected to bring in under the new system, and my name was the label under the lowest value. This was in part due to the fact I wasn't a journalist and that they also didn't believe I had the capabilities to write good stories. Somehow they'd not factored in any of the previous successes that mostly eclipsed all the 'trained people's' articles in terms of page views which they were always so desperate for.

My boss, while disturbingly smirking at me, then delivers the killer blow, "Don't get paranoid or sensitive about this, Rachael, but you're a bad writer."

He tried to justify his comment based on the fact I hadn't written a weather report in long form, because I didn't want to bore people to tears. Unless you personally spend 20 minutes reading what the weather is going to look like today, when you've a life to get on with?

You know when people give you frank yet life-changing advice that actually makes you stronger, and helps you to be better? This wasn't one of those times. Not with him sat there holding back a fit of laughter as he tore my ability to shreds. He was enjoying every minute of criticising me, and it was beyond odd. My line manager in the room didn't come to my defence either, despite stopping me to praise my style of work just a few days prior. I wanted the world to swallow me up.

We're in written form at the minute but let's pretend we've stepped into the world of film. The scene flashes back to my childhood.

When I was seven, a court order was put in place that prevented me from having any contact with my father. Although, I was told that writing letters to him would still be permitted.

We had a typewriter, but it never worked properly, so I took pen to paper and learned how to construct my sentences beyond the basics we had been taught at school. I knew I had to make it count. It was also the only way I had of expressing how I felt about the situation too.

My brother embodied the late Charles Dickens with his style, once scrawling on a postcard at the tender age of ten, "Dear Dad, I am lying here writhing in agony!" after grazing his leg following a minor skirmish with a go-kart on holiday in Tenerife.

However, something seemed to click with me. I found crafting pieces of writing made the world make sense and it was also a really good output. Not just for my own situation, but for what was happening in the world around me too.

Letters to my local MP followed, calling for action to be taken on a notoriously dangerous road where a family friend had lost her life. At one point, the Downing Street emblem poked its way through my letterbox. It was a personal response from the then prime minister Tony Blair on another issue I'd raised. All of this before the age of twelve.

I did play The Sims and eat copious amounts of candy like 'normal' kids in between trying to raise attention to various social issues that were going on around me, I should add. I just wanted to make a difference, i.e. how these journalists had also strived to do that I looked up to and had read with great intrigue as I continued to grow up.

My enthusiasm for all things words didn't go unnoticed. One teacher moved me up from one of the lower ability levels to the top set for English. I was the only kid in the year that happened to. A girl I'd previously been friends with announced how I wasn't smart enough to be in this new higher class with her, as this "was the class for future solicitors and lawyers" like her. Not people like me, coming from a single-parent family without any wealth. I got an A in that class, by the way.

Not everyone believed in my ability, of course. I was called up to see the teacher many a time because they thought I'd copied my homework directly from the internet, struggling to comprehend that I actually wrote it until I repeated it back to them word for word. My headteacher was also keen to reiterate that kids like me would not do well in life "because we hadn't been raised by both parents and that we would probably not escape the level of deprivation that we'd been born into." His thick Glaswegian accent and piercing sapphire eyes that peered over his thinly framed spectacles as he read us passages from his life-affirming book collection in school assemblies only sought to emphasise the macabre.

Ironically, it was around this age that I had started reading the publication for which I was sitting in front of the boss of at that precise moment, who was telling me I couldn't write. When they'd been publishing my work for years without even realising it, even as a child in the adult 'viewpoint' section, as I had been writing under different pseudonyms. I'd do it to test whether they thought my writing was good enough to publish, and look at what parts they'd edited so I could learn from it.

I'm mentally back in the room. I realise his comment was merely another attack on me to try and finally break me, and no, I wasn't going to let him ruin writing for me, as I had allowed so many other teachers to do over the years. You know, the ones who tell you you'll never be a success in a certain subject, as if they ever were themselves. It had happened to me in art class, music and graphic design over the years. These fuckers weren't taking my writing as well.

Raising my eyebrow to the same acute angle of that of Gene Wilder in that meme we've all seen a thousand times, I thought, do carry on. If you must.

I was then told that from now on, I would be focusing more on live blogs because I was clearly "better suited to only writing in short sentences."

Only, it wasn't feasible for me to stop writing articles for them when we had to churn out so much content in a day. We'd often need so much the management would write pieces and put others bylines on them. Sometimes the stories would be really inflammatory or general clickbait tripe, and you'd get hate for them online even though you didn't know anything about it until people tagged you in the comments.

Oh, and by the way, when they published a list of top stories at the end of that year based on work I had already done before that meeting happened, I identified the top story of the year. The third top story was mine. The fifth top story was a combination of mine and my colleague's work. This is out of thousands of articles we collectively wrote per year. Stories that broke records for page views, shares and engagement that I had direct involvement in.

I was probably on my last thread of this job, trying to hold it together, knowing that nobody at the top believed in me and drowning in criticism. I wrote an awareness piece about a common medical condition that can quickly cause death if not treated promptly. I mentioned two examples of local cases we had previously published, including a baby who had died from the condition. I was reading a difficult to decipher font, which led me to make a typo in the child's name when it was published.

Not helped by the lack of sleep and my GERD symptoms either, I must say.

Stories go through one of several editors before they are published, but the error was not picked up. Worst still, nobody warned me that, unlike other families I'd worked with who had lost children to certain conditions and welcomed the opportunity to share their story, this family was very much anti-press. Again, this was not picked up during the editing stage.

When the story went to print, I was met with a barrage of abuse from the family, who were absolutely horrified that I had mentioned her child in a recap of local cases we had published before. The worst was the mother telling me I had "disrespected the grave of their dead child" - even though I explained I had featured their case alongside others as a wider awareness piece.

I felt horrific. I had written it very respectfully, bar that regretful typo which was also due to the stress I was under and the symptoms I was experiencing health wise. But the emails from the family kept coming in their droves, and now they were focusing all of their grief - which now was apparent was still incredibly raw - onto me, almost as if I was to blame for the death of their child.

Without a doubt, all of the stories involving the death or abuse of children affected me the worst, as you can probably imagine. Given there isn't any training to deal with any of the information you will be presented with nor support afterwards, there's little wonder.

One incident that particularly stands out is a young girl who the publication had previously featured because she had gone through childhood cancer. Shortly after recovering, she was killed walking to school after being involved in a horrific road accident. An example of how life can be bitterly cruel at times.

I answered the phone a few minutes after news of this incident had been published. It was one of her relatives who didn't like how the story had been reported by my colleague. I absorbed every molecule of her grief. Yet you are in the middle of the workday with endless tasks to do, sitting in an office full of people. What can you do, especially when the other person is experiencing the worst moment of their life? I am not a trained counsellor, I am a content writer. I do not know how to help either the caller in extreme distress nor myself.

Through the shock and grief, you become someone they can essentially blame for what's happened, even if they don't realise they are effectively doing so. But how can you tell them that as if you are somehow now the victim? You can't.

I knew I had no other choice than to internalise it since that progress meeting had gone so badly, and I didn't want yet another reason for them to share their disappointment in me by admitting I was struggling.

It's funny that the ability not to feel anything, whether it be physical pain or mental anguish, is often depicted as a sign of strength, whether it be in the corporate world or even in movies. Yet, if we weren't supposed to feel pain in whatever form it takes, our bodies wouldn't have given us the ability to. We feel these signs not because we are 'weak' like we've been conditioned to believe, rather because our body is telling us enough. The question is, do we ever listen?

As you can imagine, I had full-blown GERD at this point, i.e. I wasn't eating properly, I couldn't swallow anything, and I had a searing level of heat coming from my abdomen. The medication to 'reduce my stomach acid' wasn't helping. I wasn't sleeping, and when I did sleep, I'd grind my teeth, with the number one cause of teeth grinding (bruxism) being stress and anxiety, by the way.

So, I'd go home after my shift and try to decompress. Then I'd get a phone call telling me about a new story I immediately needed to cover from home because, of course, news is 24/7 and we were only a small team. I even once got a call from a colleague on my personal rather than work phone telling me there had been a brutal murder I needed to immediately cover. At the time, I was 100 miles away from the office on a shopping trip - ironically, a trip I'd taken trying to relax from my work situation. He was apologetic when he realised I wasn't on shift, but the stress and anxiety had already washed over me and I couldn't switch off from work mode for the rest of the day.

What happens when there aren't enough staff in particular is that everyone has to be on it all the time. It could be a murder, suicide attempt, a serious accident, you name it.

For those who have prolonged exposure to trauma and stress (i.e. journalists, first responders, caregivers etc.), this can lead to a condition called compassion fatigue, which is a diminished ability to feel empathy for others. It is actually considered a secondary form of post-traumatic stress disorder because the mind is simply not able to digest further trauma, so it kind of shuts itself off almost as a protective measure.

I wonder if actually most of us have this to some degree, especially with the amount of bad news we all read on a daily basis. On the lighter end of the scale, this is known as doomscrolling. But if you're actually in the thick of that bad news every day, it's no wonder that it has a negative impact on your ability to function like a normal, caring human being. We lose the ability to feel as we should.

The problem is, I did care, and in an environment where horrific stories are your bread and butter, this is bad news. The mental and physical symptoms I was experiencing was my body's way of telling me it was overloaded, and my GERD symptoms at this point had just exploded.

I had also developed debilitating migraines at the top of my skull. My neck had lost range of motion due to a really terrible desk setup that caused a herniated disc. Plus, I didn't dare get up or leave on time, meaning I was spending far too long hunched over my desk in the most uncomfortable office chair known to man than I should have been.

It's perhaps no wonder then that poor posture is also becoming an epidemic too. Poor posture in itself can also induce GERD symptoms, in case you didn't know. Being chained to your desk for hours, especially with overtime, means your muscles get overworked, and they start to try and compensate each other, which causes painful imbalances. It can also put pressure on your organs, including the ones that digest your food.

I saw a chiropractor and physiotherapist to help me with my neck pain caused by my desk setup. My chiropractor said to me quite bluntly that this job was really affecting my health, not least my spine and that I should quit to prevent any further damage to my discs. First my mental health, then my stomach, now my spine? What the hell was going to be next?

Unable to eat, sleep or think clearly anymore I reached breaking point. I wrote a letter detailing everything I thought about the treatment of staff at the company and how it had affected my health. I handed it in with my resignation the next day. I was blunt and I was rude which is not like me.

Let me be clear here. When people spectacularly quit their jobs, they don't feel the euphoria or pride you might expect. It actually felt absolutely horrendous because all I could think about was how I was going to make everyone else's workload increase because they'd be even more short-staffed.

I stated that I was leaving the role due to the effects it was having on my mental and physical health. Aside from the required admin, nobody else reached out to me from the company, i.e. HR or higher management, to ask why I quit my job, and I never heard from my boss again.

Ironically, had we had such correspondence from any other industry, such as when we received a whistleblowing letter from a nurse detailing the working conditions at the local hospital (yes, that same one!), we would have been all over it. But, it's not as easy to hold the mirror up to their own organisation, in fact, they race to find a rug big enough to sweep what you're saying under it.

I had a notice period to work, so I consulted my doctor for advice, knowing if I went back to that office, my health was in serious jeopardy. This time, I was seen by a different doctor than my usual GP. Expecting a stern, unsympathetic response for quitting my job, having explained the situation, this new doctor stated that I was "brave and powerful" for deciding to put my health first and was extremely supportive of my decision. I could not be more grateful for the strength this gave me because it finally felt like I was being listened to. It was suggested that the disc problem in my neck had made the symptoms of my thoracic outlet syndrome worse, and so this is what ended up being used on my sick note so that I didn't have to go back rather than my GERD. FYI, three years of occipital headaches followed from that disc problem, so no it wasn't a cop out.

Of course, I was warned by my line manager the sick pay I'd be put on to cover my notice would only be about £100 a week. I didn't care about the money. I cared about my health which you cannot put a price on.

I took the time to write each of my colleagues a note and leave it on their desk. In particular, I wanted to apologise to my colleague who I was supposed to shadow to reduce his workload. I felt so bad because he'd been really kind to me and had helped me so much along the way. He was and is one of the most talented writers I've ever met, and it was a privilege that he edited my work because whenever he would oversee my work instead of my boss, he'd put an exquisite polish on my articles that was no doubt instrumental in their success when published online. He also wouldn't be afraid to pull me up when I needed to improve on something in a very fair way, and I always appreciated this as a writer. The experience of working with this particular colleague was everything I wanted the job to be. If only it could have stopped at that.

The worst part is you know it doesn't matter. You've instantly lost their respect for ditching the team when they needed you, especially when you cannot control the narrative when you're no longer physically present to defend yourself.

I came in on a Sunday and handed all my stuff back. For some reason, I also left them a cake. I don't know why I did that, but I think I was absolutely wracked with guilt because I knew how hard they all worked, and I felt like I had let them down massively. Notice how I left to protect my health on medical advice based on the impossible setup of the job, yet I was still blaming myself?

Only, I know for a fact that my perception of me at my old job probably couldn't have been further from that. I read a quote the other day that sums it up perfectly: "Don't let people manipulate you into thinking you gave up on them when you really left to save yourself."

How true is this sentiment, though? When you are ground down to such a point, you can't take it anymore, you get out for our own wellbeing. Yet, you'll still blame yourself, even though your mind and body were merely reacting to what you were being exposed to.

I was barely eating due to GERD, I now had debilitating occipital headaches, and my neck lost range of motion. Considering how excited I had been to start that job and that I had genuinely pictured a long career there, it pains me to say that there is not an inch of regret that I got out. Only that I wish I had done so sooner.

1.5 MY GERD RECOVERY

When you've experienced a sudden shift in your life, whether it be a change in job, a relationship breakdown or any other major life event that gives you a massive jolt, do you allow whatever it is to drag you down, or do you become determined that it will be the making of you?

With no job, severe GERD and now a disc problem in my neck causing me agony and triggering extremely nasty occipital headaches, it's safe to say that the odds were very much against me.

While I was incredibly humbled by what that doctor had said about my decision to quit my job, I felt where my GERD is concerned that I wanted to avoid medical intervention from this point on. I appreciate in the UK at least, our healthcare system has been overstretched for quite some time now, which could have explained why my condition was never fully explained to me, nor a healing strategy given.

Doctors frown on you doing your own research, but I had tried and tried again for someone to explain what the problem was in my stomach and, more importantly, how I could heal myself. I practically pleaded with them to give me a diet plan, but they simply shrugged their shoulders. Incredibly, not one doctor (including private treatment) ran me through what GERD was, despite prescribing me medication for it.

So I knew I had to fix this myself. I'm not saying that this avenue will be correct for everyone, but from what I can gather, GERD even baffles the medical profession, especially as there is no unified cause nor treatment. From a personal perspective, I did not get on with GERD medication. I am delighted for those who find GERD medication does work for them, but sadly this doesn't seem to be the case for most sufferers.

It's easy to think of stress as a purely mental health condition. However, stress can also create physical changes in the body, including GERD. It can also lead to things such as heart attacks, strokes and more worrying than that, even premature death if left unchecked.

However, even if the stress element is removed, the physical change often requires a similar physical approach to healing. This is why a diet plan was in order to heal the physical changes that had occurred to my stomach as a result of chronic stress.

Luckily, I had planned a return trip to California. When I got there, this really gave me time to release my stress and continue to discover new recipes and foods that had healing properties. I cannot tell you how exposure to sunshine, walks along the beach and access to highly nutritious food made me actually take notice of my health and wellbeing in a way I never really did before. It was also the first time in ages that I felt at peace.

From this point onwards, I wanted to continue to listen to my mind and body in regards to my healing strategy. It came down to the simple fact of deciphering what was going to make me feel better and what was going to make me feel worse.

Aside from the psychological causes of GERD flaring up my symptoms which I had now taken care of by leaving my job, I thought specifically about what foods made me feel worse. When I had visited California the first time while I was still really sick, one of the only meals I ate, having mostly abstained from food due to the pain, was this tomato-based pasta dish. I took about three bites, and it was like I had swallowed fire.

I remember I had to leave the restaurant because I felt really unwell. I wanted to curl up in a ball and scream. So I took some of the antacid tablets I had bought at the airport. Well, that was like adding washing detergent to the flames! I have no idea what the hell happened, as normally I found the liquid version okay. Similar to when I took omeprazole with antacids, it felt as if my stomach was bone dry and the heat was unbearable.

This gave me an epiphany. If the problem was supposed to be too much acid and I took acid reducing medication that made me feel worse, how does that work? This was the first time that it dawned on me that I probably didn't have 'too much acid' at all. I either had too little or weak stomach acid and so my stomach wasn't able to digest my foods properly. So when I ate acidic foods especially, it would burn because my stomach acid was too weak to handle it. Also, antacid medication would make me feel worse because it was depleting something I was actually critically low in. There was no other explanation at this point, so I decided to go with it seen as nothing else had worked at this point.

Once while studying graphic design, I had some work professionally printed. I went to collect it from the printers, and it appears someone ate their lunch over my work as a tiny bit of tomato seed got on the print. Where the tomato had come in contact with the paper, it had dissolved the ink because of its acidity. If that's what tomato can do to ink on a piece of paper, what was it doing to my GERD ridden stomach? No wonder I was in so much pain!

That's just it though. In normal circumstances, tomatoes are one of the best things for you because of their rich vitamin content. Only, if you are suffering from a condition affecting the acid in your stomach, it's like pouring vinegar onto an open wound. Similar to using a mouthwash containing alcohol when you have a mouth ulcer - normally it's good for you but right now it just causes pain.

The more I thought about it, I realised acidic foods made me feel worse, and alkaline foods made me feel better. I needed to come off acidic foods in order to heal because every time they passed through my stomach, they burned. It was also possible I may have an ulcer or inflamed tissue from a loosened LES muscle.

I wasn't to know any of this for sure because the gastroenterologist said I was 'too young' to have a camera put down my throat. So even they didn't know what they were treating! Clearly, they weren't interested in finding out either.

So, as drastic as it was, I decided to treat myself for what I thought the problem actually was, seeing as I couldn't feel any worse at this point. I did my research and looked at foods that were classed as acidic, including tomatoes, citrus fruits, processed foods etc., and I completely eliminated them from my diet.

I mostly stuck to my existing diet of chicken, spinach, mashed potato and gravy because these were all gentle on my stomach. I'd wash everything down with camomile tea, which I later learned is also alkaline, which is why I always felt like it soothed my stomach. Although I'd been on this diet while I was still in my old job, removing that intense level of daily stress by quitting my job really helped make this strategy a lot more effective. Otherwise, I could have taken those steps, but the stress affecting my stomach acid would have kept me going back to square one, so it was definitely necessary, not least for my sanity.

I also researched probiotics since that was the only thing the specialist could advise me to take, along with probiotic milk and consumed both daily.

However, I was still having regular flashbacks throughout the day and vivid dreams about stories I had worked on or things that had been said to me by my boss at night. I also continued to send news stories in when I would see them, even though I had left my job. I cannot explain why I did this, but I felt unable to switch off from any news story that would happen in front of me. Quite a few of them made front pages. To this day, I always see content and imagine it as a news story.

So while my mental health was still a work in progress, physically, I found the diet and lifestyle changes were really having a positive impact because I'd removed the stress element. Some days I would wake up feeling an immediate high because there was such a significant difference in how my stomach felt, and for me, that's the body's way of letting you know you're getting on top of the problem.

I was also lucky enough to get another job straight after I returned from California, which was only a couple of weeks after I had walked out of my job. I tried to remain as positive about the reasons why I had left during my interview because I wanted to leave it behind me. Unbelievably, the person who interviewed me told me not to worry because she knew people who had previously worked there who had experienced what I had hinted at also. I couldn't believe that.

My new job was based in a coastal area, and we were given an hour's lunch break, which was double that of my old job. I took the opportunity to breathe in the sea air each day, and I felt my symptoms get better each day with the change of environment. Best of all, I no longer feared my boss or even stepping through the front door each day. My new boss was actually a really lovely guy.

My GERD symptoms took around 18 months to fully settle down, and I think that's because, for that first year, I was still in my old job and also, I wasn't getting any of the right help. So, I would say my healing journey was really focused on the last six months when I took things into my own hands after leaving my job.

If I had known from the start about the effect of stress on the gut, plus that I actually had GERD and how to properly address it, I'm sure I could have healed much sooner. As I said, I wasn't even told which foods to eat or drink, bar the suggestion of peppermint tea which is actually a major GERD trigger. So something is clearly very wrong, given GERD and even heartburn remain extremely common conditions, yet medically it's just not being grasped in a way that brings effective healing to patients.

That is just one of the many reasons I felt it was important to make my story public because although each of you will have different reasons for developing GERD, ultimately, without information, we all end up stuck in the same miserable cycle.

Throughout the rest of the sections of this book, I will detail how I healed and, specifically, how I approached the topic of food. It is my sincere wish that this offers benefit to anyone who is experiencing GERD, especially GERD caused by stress or simply a lifestyle that is not in balance with our basic human needs.

1.6 GETTING GERD DIAGNOSED

Despite the fact I took my healing into my own hands, it's still essential to get off Google and see a doctor. I know this is tricky for those who don't have free healthcare, but it needs to happen all the same. You might find it helpful to write down all of your symptoms before you go in to avoid missing any key details.

If you have any extreme symptoms, seek medical attention immediately to rule out anything such as gallstones, appendicitis etc. You know your body better than anyone, so trust your instincts - especially if you are suddenly much worse, struggling to breathe, have chest pains etc.

Most cases of GERD are diagnosed through conversation alone. However, testing can include an upper endoscopy, where they put a camera down your throat to physically identify the problem.

An ambulatory acid (pH) probe test monitors the acid in your stomach. In the UK (and I assume elsewhere), we have a similar test called an esophageal manometry test, which is a monitor that checks if the nerves and the muscles of the stomach are functioning properly. It also checks whether the LES valve is working as it should be. I haven't seen either test talked about much in the UK, and Google leads me to a random PDF instead of the main NHS website, which is never a good sign when it comes to common use or information.

Another option is imaging of your upper abdomen, which is taken after you drink a chalky liquid, which allows the doctor to get a better picture of your esophagus.

I personally wasn't offered any investigations, other than the basic one where a doctor presses on different parts of your abdomen to check where the pain is, along with the ultrasound of my abdomen (in fairness, they had to repeat it four times because they didn't know how to read the images!). So, if I could do things differently in the form of advising anyone reading this, it would be to push for the tests you feel you need.

I did some research, and endoscopies are only recommended for patients above 45 with GERD symptoms. I have to say I find this obscene, and I sincerely hope this changes. Just FYI, you don't suffer any less with GERD depending on how old you are. It still deserves the same level of medical care whether you're 25 or 75.

The reason I wanted the camera investigation is that if I bent forward later in the day to pick something up or try to exercise less than four hours after last eating, I would develop a flare-up. I never used to have this growing up, even when I would go to gymnastics right after eating dinner where I was doing bar work hanging upside down or vaulting. From what I've read, bending forward increases the amount of stomach acid that can get into the esophagus. So, there's definitely something at play here.

Coincidently, I had an unrelated MRI for my thoracic outlet syndrome, and it found I have an aberrant right subclavian artery. In short, the right subclavian artery travels off the heart and supplies the right arm with blood. Only mine deviates and wraps around my esophagus. I'm sorry, I feel like we've sashayed into an episode of House here, but stay with me.

My vascular surgeon advised it wouldn't cause me too much of an issue unless I had my trachea cut, and the surgeon wasn't aware, as they'd cut through this vital artery accidentally, and I'd bleed to death. How jolly. Other than that, GERD wasn't mentioned as a possible side effect. Though a quick bit of Googling has told me an aberrant right subclavian artery could cause symptoms for both TOS and GERD. But what are you supposed to think when a qualified surgeon tells you it's unrelated and 'not to worry'? It's so confusing and honestly just exhausting to think about. I have healed now, so I'll trust his opinion on that, but it's an interesting theory nonetheless for anyone in a similar boat.

I should warn you, you're probably going to get misdiagnosed. The further up the chain you get in your healthcare plan, the more you are likely to be patronised. I'm hopeful that this won't be everyone's experience, but I can only go on my own, and that of my followers telling me exactly the same stories. What is going on here?

Even though I have gotten better of my own accord, I would still advise pushing for the investigations you want, or at least getting a second opinion. I know a lot of people feel too shy to do this, but it's your body at the end of the day. You need to know what's up with it. Nobody has a right to tell you otherwise.

1.7 GERD: WHY THERE'S NO EASY WAY OUT

The frustrating thing about GERD is that symptoms can show up suddenly, yet getting rid of the condition takes a sustained effort that might take weeks or months to start to fix.

Don't panic. You will learn everything you need that is of value in this book otherwise, I wouldn't have bothered writing it. That said, I've spent a fair bit of time answering comments on my GERD videos and reading posts on social media sites, and I seem to come across the same patterns, i.e. **everyone is looking for that magic cure.** To be able to pop just one pill and never hear from your GERD again, and of course to guzzle that bucket of fried chicken afterwards with no repercussions.

Only fixing GERD doesn't work like that because your body isn't stupid. Even reading this book alone won't help you if you don't take away any of the steps and actually make a conscious effort to change your habits.

I've been there, I know that when you're at your lowest ebb, it's horrendous. It goes on for days, weeks, months and for some poor folks years. So the only way you're going to heal is to commit to the cause, bearing in mind your personal GERD triggers and looking at how your overall health and wellbeing are faring.

Hence the emphasis needs to move away on looking for an overnight cure. If you take your healing seriously and really commit to it (including identifying your personal causes/triggers), then things will improve. To be honest, nothing can be as bad as staying as ill as you are, so please give yourself a break here and get real with your expectations.

Healing Time Frame - How Long Does It Take To Heal From GERD?

People frequently contact me to ask how long it will take them to heal from GERD. Bearing in mind, I am not a doctor, I know nothing about them personally, their GERD cause or even their personal triggers.

I get it. We all want definite answers, especially against the backdrop of so much uncertainty, and let's be honest, pain and misery. But, I think it's a problem when we look to solely focus on time frames rather than the steps we should be actively concentrating on.

I had mentioned in my video and in this book that when I finally understood the condition, it took me around six months to get to a point where I could eat and drink most foods again without issue. This followed a year of my GERD going untreated properly and an origin of stress which then caused physical problems with my digestion. Your condition may be more severe than mine, which could take longer to heal, or less severe, which may take less time to heal.

Similar to asking a personal trainer at the gym how long it will take to get a six-pack, no two people will be given the same answer because it depends on their current shape, what methods they adopt and ultimately whether they are committed or not.

Needless to say, **your GERD isn't going to disappear overnight** because that's impossible. But I am aiming to get you feeling better within a matter of weeks and back to your old self as soon as possible. If you can't commit fully, then this process will be delayed, which is why although I am giving you the information that helped me, the onus is on you to follow it.

So, I want you to simply focus on putting your all into healing based on what I am explaining as a former GERD patient because if you do so diligently enough, the rest will follow.

I also want you to shift the focus of your healing off of what I can do for you (when giving a timeframe is something I simply cannot do for you personally) onto what you can do for yourself.

I am also assuming you have visited a doctor to ensure it's definitely GERD you are dealing with and that it isn't due to an anatomical defect or hormonal cause, but that it is diet or stress related. So get your ducks in a row, and let's focus on what we can control.

1.8 PREPARING YOURSELF FOR CHANGE

In this modern world, we worship material things and even celebrities on social media. When in reality, the most precious thing we should actually be concentrating on is our health.

I know most people hate change. It's not that they hate it per se, it's that change forces us to act or think differently. To make an effort and to challenge ourselves. To confront what we keep burying. So, if you are looking for that 'easy' way out with GERD, let me be clear it doesn't exist. Though, you can consider a lot of these changes easy given they are things you can do for free without spending the earth. Some changes are even what's going on inside your head!

If you're making changes to improve your GERD, especially if yours is diet or mental health related, then you can't underestimate how huge this is going to be. Of course, change is needed because if you keep as you are, it's clearly not going to make you feel better.

When you know precisely what your GERD triggers are, and they are something that's fixable, then you're either committed to fixing them, or you're not. That's not to say you won't have ups and downs because you will. But equally, you can't really make a half-arsed attempt and expect miracles here.

Ultimately, there's no escaping that recovering from GERD is going to take a lot of changes with regards to what you eat and how you take care of yourself in general. The problem is change is just not that easy regardless of what your goal is.

The key takeaway here is that unhealthy food is addictive. As with any addiction, quitting 'just like that' is basically impossible because our brains have become hard-wired to crave that bucket of chicken or big ol' bowl of ice cream.

Furthermore, the reason you make poor dietary choices or smoke isn't just because you're addicted - it can be down to a lack of education on the health implications and even more common than that because you are using it as a coping mechanism. As was I, by eating chocolate at work every time I felt stressed. So, unless you get to the root cause of why you eat certain foods or light up a cigarette when you are stressed, you'll continue to not be able to give these things up.

The problem also is that we try to go from one extreme to the other. Take New Year's resolutions as an example. You have this massive blowout over Christmas where you eat and drink everything in sight. Then Suddenly, on January 1st, you expect to be able to survive on a 3-day juice cleanse. All it does is shock your body, make you hangry (angry because you're hungry), and well, it's a recipe for failure. Instead, it needs to be a gradual switch to a healthier diet and lifestyle. Otherwise, you'll be back to where you started in no time.

There are also possible psychological issues with vegetables that stem from childhood. Think about kids when they are taken to a fast food restaurant. They enjoy that food because the experience is fun, and in some places, they even get a free toy. But when they sit down to a plate of vegetables, the tone changes. They are told to 'get it eaten' whether they like what's on the plate or not. Or that they aren't leaving the table until their plate is cleared.

Sometimes, parents will inadvertently create a controlling, negative experience that will be with the child for the rest of their life. So as adults, they keep away from vegetables in response. The brain automatically makes that connection with stress release through eating crap food. Like I've said before, nobody goes through a breakup and then immediately orders a salad.

So if any of this resonates with you (especially if you had any negative experiences with food as a child) then you may need to take the time to rediscover certain fruits and vegetables. It's not about forcing yourself to eat what you really, really hate either. More, trying to move away from past negative experiences around food that without you even realising it could be stopping you from making nutritional progress as an adult.

Given so many of the foods that cause GERD are processed or unhealthy, it's at least worth considering. If you're unsure, consult a nutritionist or therapist to get to the root cause of your dislike for healthy food. I promise it will be well worth the investment.

Every Day Is A Clean Slate

Each day we are lucky enough to wake up to is a chance to hit the reset button on our health. But, the majority of people continue as they are. Don't be the person who ignores warning signs their body gives them.

Think about your first meal of the day. Sure, you could opt for a fried bacon sandwich. But what is that actually going to do to your body?

If I suggest having a green smoothie or a bowl of oatmeal with healthy seeds instead, you'll either be someone who thinks, 'yeah, I'm up for that!' or 'hell no'. If you belong to the latter group, you can hardly complain if chronic illness sets in because as tasty as junk food might be, it's not what nature intended for us to eat - especially if you're eating it in copious amounts.

The ironic thing is that doctors will likely give out medication to try and counteract the effects of eating crap foods such as tablets to reduce cholesterol or blood pressure, when most people could fix everything all on their own for free, if they just treated tomorrow as a clean slate.

Whether you're dealing with GERD or any other condition, just stop and think for a second before you shove these things into your body. Make the connection between the food and drink you consume and your health.

1.9 DEALING WITH HOPELESSNESS

As I alluded to at the start of this book, something that isn't well acknowledged with any chronic health condition is that when it's causing you a lot of distress, it's been going on for a while, and you aren't getting anywhere with treating it, the mental health implications can be huge. You also might not have anyone you can talk to about it because you don't want to burden those around you, or your circle simply doesn't understand.

I've also noticed support groups on social media aren't beneficial either for a few reasons. Firstly, you get constant updates and notifications about your condition, meaning it's tough to switch off from it. Sometimes, you're having a really great day, and you see people writing they can't carry on because they have your condition. These people obviously need a great deal of support, but by posting such content, it's so easy to pull others down who are also struggling, especially when, even during their downtime, they are constantly reminded they have the same thing. It's an overload.

The second reason is I often find social media groups to be a bit of an echo chamber. For example, someone will post they need advice about something. The thread will get 20 responses of people talking in the first person, not even acknowledging a single thing the original poster has said. How is that person able to get support when everyone replying is using it as an excuse to talk about themselves?

That's why I told my followers I was writing this book, and I said to them, tell me everything you want me to cover. I made sure every point was a chapter so that people who need help find value in what I'm saying. Otherwise, how can I help someone if I don't listen to what they are asking? This book might be my story, but it's about helping you.

Not all support groups are like this, and you can definitely find some helpful information out there. But I'd advise caution spending too much time engaging in reading anything which will depress you about your condition rather than spurring you on to treat it because it's such an easy black hole to fall down when you're struggling.

Sometimes we actually have too much information at our fingertips. I went through a period of health anxiety a few years ago, and the ability to Google every finding on an MRI report really doesn't help. There's an invisible line between informing yourself and scaring yourself to death. The worst thing you can do when you're going through a health battle is cross that line. So beware.

So what should you do when you are having a down day? Well firstly, don't eat or drink anything that is going to make it worse, that's a given. I have a whole section on camomile tea coming up, and spoiler alert I'm going to be telling you to go make a cup of it right now. Go on pause, my words will wait, they are printed using good ink. At least that's what I'm assuming Amazon's commission is spent on, anyway!

What you need to do is find something you really enjoy that won't aggravate your condition, whether this is watching a comedy show, spending time with friends, even playing a good old game of cards. Basically, anything you enjoy which will not induce your stress levels or cause you anatomically to have a flare-up of your GERD. I challenge you to write down ten things now, store the list in your phone and come back to it when you're feeling low.

It's also ok to get upset sometimes. I know it doesn't feel nice, but sometimes you have to release that pent up emotion of trying to pretend you're ok when you're not. A lot of people feel much better for doing so.

I definitely had those moments myself, especially after the blood incident. I was really worried I wasn't going to beat this, but in the end, I did, and there's no reason why you can't either, especially if your condition is definitely GERD and you take the steps that myself and others who have recovered offer to you. I didn't have that, I figured everything out as I went along, which was very lonely at times.

I posted a video on my channel about my struggles and received thousands of comments from people going through exactly the same thing. Most of my videos have a few hundred views, so I never expected so many people to resonate with me. Especially not to the point where I'm sitting writing a book about the whole experience! So remember, you aren't alone at all.

You're also going to have days where you feel a bit better, then have a crap day. With any medical condition, there are always going to be highs and lows, even if you're on the path to recovery. If that's where you're at now, then don't beat yourself up. It doesn't mean you aren't going to get through it. Instead, you just need to get better at listening to your triggers.

I'll be honest, people around you might not want to hear about your difficulties. They might not be very supportive or offer the right advice because they can't sympathise with you. But, any other conversations you can have with them are still helpful. Maybe not when you really need to talk to someone who understands, but still, don't cut yourself off when you are going through something this challenging. Even a generic chat about the weather is better than a wall of silence with only your pain for company.

2.0 MY EXPERIENCE WITH GERD MEDICATION

When your doctor suspects you have GERD or heartburn, you will likely be offered medication to try to relieve your symptoms.

Some of the main medications used to treat GERD include lansoprazole, omeprazole, esomeprazole, pantoprazole, rabeprazole and dexlansoprazole, which are known as proton pump inhibitors (PPI) that are designed to block acid production.

In cases where a loosening of the LES muscle is thought to be to blame for your symptoms,
baclofen may be prescribed as it's thought to decrease the level of relaxation in the valve that allows the stomach acid to flow upwards into your throat.

I was put on omeprazole which is a proton pump inhibitor, and told to take antacid medication after eating. You may have noticed that the 2.0 section of this book is rather short, and that's because I followed the instructions diligently, but I couldn't understand why not only was this medication not helping me, but it would make me feel much worse, to the point where I would absolutely dread taking it because of the searing pain that would follow.

In fact, having moderated some 2,000 comments on my GERD

video up to now, not one single person has told me that GERD medication genuinely helped them. While I cannot personally advise anyone on what medication to take or not to take, it stands to reason that if you've tried GERD medication and it hasn't helped you, it's probably not the right approach; hence, why you're probably reading this book.

It was probably my third visit to the doctor, which saw me being prescribed omeprazole, which is designed to relieve the symptoms of GERD, in addition to repairing damage caused by the stomach acid entering the esophagus (erosive esophagitis).

When I would take omeprazole, I would feel my stomach dry up. Considering what we just went over with the fact your stomach can have too much or indeed too little acid, I strongly suspect my acid was depleted. Because I cannot understand why, when I'd take omeprazole, let alone antacids, it would leave me feeling worse. *Much much worse.* The only explanation is that either omeprazole leaves everyone feeling like that - in which case, why would it be so commonly prescribed? Or could it be that in my particular case, my stomach acid was on the low side? So, when I felt the antacids and omeprazole 'dry out' my stomach creating even more discomfort, I wasn't imagining it?

Do you know that relief you get when you're prescribed something that genuinely takes the pain off or relieves your symptoms? I never got that with omeprazole. The only way I can describe it is like having an Indian burn but to your internal organs. Now yes, I was still in a stressful environment which wasn't helping at the time. But surely, if it was the right medication for what was specifically going on with my body, I would have felt at least some easing of my symptoms? All it did was make me feel worse.

Another problem I have with omeprazole is, like all medications, we get lured into a false sense of security that whatever is going wrong with our bodies can be fixed merely by taking a pill.

Now in some cases, omeprazole absolutely does work, and this is fantastic. If this is you, I'm really happy for you. But it wasn't the case for me, nor has it helped those commenting on my video who are also noting that it only made them feel worse. Believe me, I take no joy in this, and I wish I didn't have to be trying to provide the answers here, especially as a patient and not as a doctor.

No, that doesn't mean I'm telling you not to take omeprazole or to stop taking any medication you have been prescribed. That has to be a decision between you and your doctor. If you're taking it now, and it's working, then why would you stop taking it? The thing I'm talking about is when medication is really not helping; in fact, it's making you feel worse, especially when you've been taking it for some time, and there's still no relief. These are completely different scenarios.

Either way, the sooner you come to terms with healing yourself of any ailment can never be down to a pill alone, the easier time you will have with things, especially when you start to apply that mindset to the actions you take in everyday life.

For example, there are genuinely people out there who think they can take omeprazole and other antacids that work for them and then guzzle down a greasy burger and several pints of alcohol straight after. Oh, and head out for a smoke after they are done. It just doesn't work like that, and you know it.

Then there are the side effects of omeprazole that nobody ever talks about. These aren't mere rumours; I'm citing actual BMJ publications and studies. In their report, 'The Understated Dangers of Omeprazole' published January 2000, the author starts off by saying, "there are many serious adverse physiological effects that occur routinely with this drug." Pardon the pun, but gulp.

To summarise, they found that taking omeprazole can cause

B12 deficiency or malabsorption, the effects of which can be irreversible. This is in addition to decreased gastric emptying rate, which means your stomach will empty at a slower rate. Also, the report stated omeprazole can cause decreased gastric ascorbic acid levels, which can trigger gastritis, aka a similar condition to GERD. Continued omeprazole use can even be carcinogenic. Please give that paper a read if you don't believe me.

Now, omeprazole is far from the only medication out there which has potential side effects, even really scary ones. Sometimes we have to take such medications because it's the only way the condition we are suffering from will get better. As an example, antibiotics kill both good and bad bacteria, which is why it's recommended you take probiotics after a course of antibiotics. It's not possible to avoid antibiotics if prescribed because they are needed for that specific problem, even if they may cause other issues as a result.

Perhaps what's needed is an honest conversation about not only the side effects of omeprazole but also how a patient can minimise the chances of complications. Whether this needs to come from the drug manufacturer or doctors, I don't know. Again, the risk of complications is why doctors are so keen to monitor you on any medication, which is yet another reason you can't dismiss their vast medical expertise, even if you're very frustrated.

PPI medication is not designed as a long term solution. In the UK, the NHS recommends not to take it for longer than two weeks without checking in with a doctor as you may require further tests or different medication. All the while, all these doctor's appointments you keep having to go to don't exactly fit with your work schedule, which is why being given medication that isn't helping when you do make it to the doctors couldn't be more frustrating.

This may or may not come as a shock, but did you know the pharmaceutical industry is the biggest industry in the world? At the time of writing, **the pharmaceutical industry is worth $1.2 trillion worldwide**. The US represents 48% of the global pharmaceutical market.

I noticed that when I used to blog about skincare, I never saw people raving about cucumber or aloe vera to treat dry skin even though it's highly effective, especially if your skin is irritated or sensitive. Then I realised there's no money to be made in doing that! I highly suspect the same has happened with the pharmaceutical industry and GERD being one of the most common health conditions has been caught up in the mix.

As I said, if omeprazole is working wonders for you and life is fantastic - keep as you are. However, as a patient, I can only go on my own personal experiences with GERD medication which were not good. My personal opinion is that I don't think you can cure GERD by popping a tablet and gulping liquid antacids. Instead, I found it has to be a more rounded approach to fixing your diet and lifestyle over the longer term.

In another recent study published by Harvard, they note that taking PPIs on a short term basis is generally considered safe. However, long term use has been linked to low levels of vitamin B12, magnesium and calcium. They also mention that some studies have linked long term PPI use with an increased risk of hip fractures, pneumonia, kidney disease, cardiovascular disease and dementia.

Now, it's worth mentioning that PPIs are not designed to be used for long periods, which is why I mentioned above here in the UK, at least they monitor you. But given such medication is freely available over the counter in many countries, there are probably a lot of people who slip through the net.

As always, I am not a doctor (though I jest that I watch a lot of House). I can't tell you from a medical perspective what is right or wrong. But, what will tell you is your body. If taking omeprazole or any other medication ISN'T helping - then that is the best indicator of all. It's not the right approach for you. But don't give up - get smart and determined to fix your health for good.

The publication from Harvard also reminds patients not to stop suddenly taking PPIs, so keep this in mind also. That's why it always pays to consult your doctor. Yes, even if you feel like you aren't getting anywhere. Just to be safe.

If you are prescribed omeprazole and you're apprehensive, monitor how you feel on it. Ask yourself if it's genuinely making you feel better, alongside other dietary and lifestyle changes you need to make. If your symptoms suddenly become much worse or do not improve, it's time to have another chat with your doctor. So wherever you are in the world, make sure someone in the medical profession is keeping an eye on you.

Furthermore, I personally would advise asking your doctor if there is another option versus taking omeprazole or antacids altogether. For instance, would your doctor allow you to try healing yourself through diet and lifestyle changes first? It's worth asking, in my opinion. If they say no and give clarification why then at least you can make an informed decision. But just handing you a pill without explaining why you've ended up this way and what you should have done differently just seems backwards if we are to encourage long term change, regardless of whether we are talking about GERD or any other health condition.

2.1 THE PINK GOO

The pink goo refers to a brand of liquid antacid medication that is readily available in most stores. It begins with 'G', and no, that doesn't stand for gut. I'm not naming the brand name in case they get a bit irked that I'm going to tell you not to rely on it.

A good analogy I heard about liquid antacid medication is that it's basically the equivalent of putting a lid on a volcano. So yes, it's fine as a temporary measure, just to get you out of a jam, especially after eating lunch at work. Or if you only suffer from occasional heartburn. However, it's not going to deal with the hot, volcanic raging furnace below. That can only come from changes you make to your diet and lifestyle, in addition to checking for any anatomical problems if you suspect you might have some.

The Pink Goo isn't just aimed at us GERD sufferers either. Every year at Christmas, there are several different TV adverts for antacid medications, both in liquid and tablet form. They advise you to 'stock up' so that you can indulge and enjoy the big day. In America, you might see these types of adverts more around Thanksgiving.

I'm sorry to break the bad news, but your stomach doesn't suddenly decide it can handle 4x more food, grease and alcohol just because it's a holiday. This is not me trying to be a killjoy; it's me trying to get you to imagine your internal organs once you swallow that food. If you eat too much, especially in a short space of time, all of that food has nowhere to go. Your stomach may stretch, and you can experience heartburn when your stomach acid struggles to break the food down. Why would you honestly want to eat or drink to such excess where that ends up happening?

I can tell you that the pleasure of eating whatever it was will soon disappear when you feel bloated and sick. When the contents of your stomach acid and bile are sitting in your throat.

Why do we look to The Pink Goo to 'save' us from such a fate when we could save ourselves instead?

Part of the problem is that we have these big releases of stress and life pressures during holidays. For some of you, it might even be the holidays themselves that cause you the pressure in the first place, especially if you're expected to cook, look after guests, buy presents you can't afford, spend time with family you don't get on with or whatever it may be. Some people also find holidays put what they are missing in life under a giant microscope, so it can definitely work multiple ways.

Taking this back to what you eat around the holidays, it's about making that emotional connection, which directly correlates with how we eat to suppress our feelings. I'm not for a second saying don't go out and enjoy yourself, but equally be mindful of your limit. When you feel full, don't keep pushing your stomach.

I'm also asking you to question why holidays feel like such a relief, or as the case may be a time to try and forget what's happening in your life.

Each of the reasons that just came to mind is something to work on so that when the holidays roll around, you absolutely can enjoy yourself, but not to the level where you are eating your emotions, causing GERD or heartburn as a result. Take the time to make the mental connection so that you don't have to rely on a liquid that keeps the contents of your stomach out of your esophagus. I promise you'll feel so much better for it.

2.2 MY THOUGHTS ON APPLE CIDER VINEGAR

When I was searching for a cure for my GERD I frequently came across videos where people would suggest glugging apple cider vinegar. I even bought some myself, but my gut (pardon the pun) told me not to do it. Upon further research, I found that apple cider vinegar is 2.0-3.0 on the pH scale. That puts ACV almost as strong as lemon but not quite as strong as a tomato. Given eating tomato-based foods left me in AGONY, how would drinking something EVEN MORE ACIDIC help my case?

Furthermore, the strong acidity of ACV can actually erode your tooth enamel which is why dentists do not advise people to drink it neat. Instead, they suggest watering it down. Once again, you cannot 'shock' your stomach with weird remedies to try to fix your GERD, especially if there's a huge underlying cause such as poor diet choices, stress or even a hernia you need to actually focus on.

Like I always say, if you personally feel that apple cider vinegar is the way to go - then don't let me stop you. We're all on our personal journey here. But, using common sense - consuming a highly acidic liquid when your stomach acid is already gravely struggling with the acidity of regular food and drink is not likely to end well. For those with no existing stomach issues, you're probably not going to have much of a problem so long as you don't drink it neat to protect your teeth.

I know that so many people rave about it. I've also had plenty of comments on my channel with people who are extremely offended - as if I had dissed their choice of baby name - because I didn't want to try it while I was in extreme agony. I'm not going to apologise for my personal feelings on something when this is my GERD story, you know? If you aren't experiencing GERD and enjoy adding it to your diet and have noticed no ill effects, then, of course, do as you are. It's just a whole different ball game when you have GERD, especially when it's severe.

I reiterate what I've explained before about treading lightly. Now is NOT the time for crazy dietary experiments. If you want to try apple cider vinegar as a preventative measure and you feel no ill effects, go for it. However, I strongly advise against anyone with GERD rushing in and gulping anything highly acidic, regardless of what people pushing their own agenda will tell you. Sorry!

I appreciate that it's too overcautious for some, but when every single thing leaves you in extreme discomfort, you can't be too careful. Apple cider vinegar was not a part of my healing journey, so if I tell you to go take it, then I'm not being honest with you about how I healed, and I refuse to be anything other than completely honest when this condition is so utterly miserable. After all, I've written this book to help you to get better.

3.0 EATING WITH GERD

No, the title of this section isn't a joke you find in a Christmas cracker. You really do have to learn how to eat with GERD before slowly reintroducing more foods once you feel better.

One of the most important things when it comes to GERD is not to overeat. The problem is, sometimes it feels as if you are still hungry, so you have that extra bite. Or even that extra snack after dinner. If you've been struggling to eat and you feel hungry, it can really feel tempting to go all out. Overeating will seriously flare-up your GERD, so I can't stress enough how you need to eat smaller portions and to stop eating before you get too full.

I can remember my first experience of heartburn vividly as it happens. I was five years old, and I had just started school. Back in the 90s in the UK, school dinners were the finest cuisine you could ever wish to taste (it all went downhill in the early 2000s when they introduced cold sandwiches and packs of raisins for lunch instead). Anyway, after serving you a beautiful roast dinner, you'd also get a pudding. On that day, it was a sponge dessert with royal icing, a cherry on top smothered in custard. It was that nice, I went back for seconds as they said they had plenty left if anyone wanted anymore. I'd of course overeaten by having that second helping, and I spent the rest of the day and evening feeling really full and sick.

Portion sizes, in general, are a problem. Most people eat far too much food in one sitting, which is not only bad for our waistlines, but for GERD, it will undo every bit of progress you've made so far. So you have to go easy. Even if you are eating the right food, that doesn't mean you can just stuff yourself. Instead, you have to take baby steps because your stomach is delicate right now.

The timing of when you eat is important too. Try not to eat for at least three to four hours before you go to sleep. The reason is that if your LES muscle isn't keeping the 'door' of your stomach shut and you lie down too close after eating, that acid is just going to fly straight up. It's all to do with gravity.

I used to be someone who would eat a lot of chocolate, especially after mealtimes. This is bad because sugar causes inflammation. But worse than that, chocolate, like coffee, contains methylxanthine - this actually relaxes muscles, including your all-important LES muscle. Chocolate is also high in fat! So, do yourself a favour and slowly wean yourself off sugar altogether if at all possible. I know that's a very daunting process but I promise once you kick the habit for good, you will be glad you did.

The truth is you have to think about every bite. No, not in an obsessive kind of way that could lead to an eating disorder. What I mean is, you can't afford to be carefree and shovel in junk food and candy anymore. Nor fizzy drinks or the odd cigarette. Everything that comes into contact with your stomach is either going to make or break your recovery.

Methods of eating with GERD must remain within the following:

- Eat raw (where applicable)
- Steam
- Bake
- Boil (last resort though as it reduces nutrients)

Switch to low-fat cooking oil or better still, spray which lightly coats the pan. If you're using too much oil in the pan, regardless of what you're cooking, it's going to trigger your symptoms. Your days of see-through paper bags lined with grease containing your lunch are over.

If you steam your food (i.e. veggies), then you don't even have to use anything to line a steamer, which will be even better for your recovery.

Absolutely NO frying your food, other than making something like a healthy stir fry. Even then, the food is being cooked by the fast rotation of heat rather than letting the food sit in gallons of oil.

I can remember in my new job, I once bought a green smoothie on my lunch break and brought it back to the office. A coworker came up to me just to tell me he thought my drink looked "absolutely disgusting."

The irony being, if I had brought back a burger, he probably would have told me it looked delicious, and that he now wanted one. Even though the green smoothie had natural, healthy ingredients in it that nourish the body, and a burger would have been full of crap.

Somewhere along the lines, we've gotten terribly muddled up. So throughout this next section, it's about undoing our bad habits to bring a sense of harmony to our gut, which isn't best pleased with us at the minute!

3.1 THE PH SCALE EXPLAINED

We know that with GERD, in the majority of cases, our stomach acid isn't doing so well. So, going on the basis that our stomach acid either isn't acidic enough or there isn't enough of it (as always, please identify your personal cause of GERD to be sure), the answer lies in not upsetting your stomach any further. This means that in the meantime, not consuming any foods or drinks that are more acidic than your stomach acid, nor are too much for your depleted stomach acid to be able to break down.

All of which hinge on understanding the pH scale. As we know, stomach acid can have a pH of around 1.0-3.0 when it's in its normal healthy state. Assuming the acid has weakened, making it not acidic enough is generalising GERD somewhat, though it can help anyone who is having difficulty with GERD or heartburn, so long as you don't have a hernia or are pregnant, as dietary changes may not fix your underlying cause.

So, what's the opposite of acidic? Alkaline! Anything with a pH of 6.0 and above is where we need to aim, seen as this gets us away from acids and into the neutrals before moving up to alkaline, which is pH 8.0 and above.

Below are the pH readings of various foods and drinks. As universal readings, **they may differ slightly from if you were to repeat the test.** For example, there are endless varieties of apples, and some are sweeter and others more bitter, so this will affect the pH, as will cooking food. So, I encourage you to do your own research if you're unsure.

Also, just because an item is deemed to be acidic, that doesn't mean it will specifically cause a flare-up. But, it's handy to note, especially if you are going through the worst of it, so you can avoid any potential triggers.

Likewise, I have gotten a lot of questions as to why some healthy foods such as lemon or tomato are acidic when they believe such foods have an 'alkalising effect on the body'. What I want you to picture here is that food passing directly over inflamed tissue - if it's acidic, it doesn't matter how healthy it is, it's going to burn like hell. So until your GERD symptoms simmer down, acidic foods, drinks and activities need to be avoided.

Most food and drink that are safe to eat with GERD will fall between the 7.0 and 9.0 range. Let me be clear, that's not to say you should only eat within that pH range. Try not to get too obsessed with just how alkaline a food is, just make sure it's not an **obvious acid** while you're trying to heal, and you should be grand.

There may also be some anomalies. For example, some foods that are acid you may be perfectly ok with. Likewise, some alkaline foods may trigger you. So, don't take it as absolute gospel, but use the pH scale as a general guide. See how **you personally react** and make a note of anything that doesn't agree with you.

P.S: I printed this book in black and white to reduce printing costs that would have been passed on to you, but it may help to get some coloured pens or crayons and shade in the colours of the pH scale below. For example, red is acidic, green is neutral, and purple is alkaline. You could even get super fancy and colour code all 12 shades!

0 ---- Severely Acidic

1 ---- Extremely Acidic

2 ---- Very Acidic

3 ---- Quite Acidic

4 ---- Fairly Acidic

5 ---- Moderately Acidic

6 ---- Slightly Acidic

7 ---- Neutral

8 ---- Slightly Alkaline

9 ---- Moderately Alkaline

10 ---- Fairly Alkaline

11 ---- Quite Alkaline

12 ---- Very Alkaline

13 ----Extremely Alkaline

14 ---- Severely Alkaline

Drinks	Typical pH
Apple cider vinegar	2.0 - 3.0
Apple juice	3.0 - 4.50
Beer	4.0 - 5.0

Black tea	4.9 - 5.50
Camomile tea	**7.0**
Carbonated water	3.0 - 4.0
Carrot juice	**6.20 - 7.0**
Celery juice	**5.70 - 6.0**
Cider	3.20 - 3.60
Coconut Water	5.0 - 5.40
Coffee	4.85 - 5.10
Cola (diet)	3.20
Cola (regular)	2.30
Cranberry juice	2.60
Energy drinks	2.52 - 3.81
Ginger ale	2.0 - 4.0
Grape juice	3.0 - 4.0
Lemon juice	2.0 - 2.60
Lime juice	2.0 - 3.50
Milk	**6.50 - 6.70**
Oat Milk	**6.70 - 6.90**
Orange juice	3.30 - 4.20

Pineapple juice	3.50 - 5.20
Prune juice	5.0
Rum	4.80
Tequila	3.20
Tomato juice	4.05 - 4.65
Water	**7.0**
Wine (red)	3.30 - 3.60
Wine (white)	3.10 - 3.40

Notes:

Celery juice is thought to restore hydrochloric acid and bile production. It's not the best tasting thing in the world, but if you can 'stomach' it for want of a better phrase, consuming neat every morning 30 minutes before food is recommended by experts.

Milk can be a trigger for some due to it being a dairy product. In addition, some milk is high in fat. Switch to plant-based milk such as almond or oat if you notice cow's milk triggers your symptoms.

Water quality is going to differ depending on where you live. Make sure your water is safe to drink. You may also want to invest in a water filter or purifier.

Now do you understand why that cup of coffee or alcoholic spirit burns so much? It's acidic.

On the other end of the scale, you'll notice how camomile tea has a pH of between 6.0 and 7.0. Now, 6.0 is just on the cusp of neutral, and 7.0 is neutral. The drink is also filled with water and without milk, sugar or sweeteners meaning the water will neutralise it further.

If you really want to be on the safe side, loose camomile may work out more alkaline but either way, I can assure you either way camomile tea is excellent for GERD. It's also possible the water you use may affect the acidity, so go for filtered or bottled water if your local tap water isn't of good quality (please recycle any plastic you use if you have to use bottled water). Even though tap water usually scores highly on the alkaline scale, it really depends on your specific location.

I have highlighted all the foods I personally have found to be GERD friendly, including any anomalies, whereby the pH is on the lower side, yet does not cause me to have a flare-up. Feel free to cross out any foods you do not find to be GERD friendly as part of your personal healing journey.

Vegetables	Typical pH
Artichokes (Jerusalem)	**5.93 - 6.0**
Asparagus	**6.0 - 7.0**
Aubergine (eggplant)	4.50 - 5.30
Avocado	**6.27 - 6.58**
Bamboo shoots	5.65

Beetroot	5.30 - 6.60
Black beans	5.78 - 6.02
Broccoli	6.41
Brussels sprout	6.15
Cabbage (green)	6.13
Cabbage (red)	5.80
Cabbage (savoy)	6.30
Cabbage (white)	6.20
Carrots	6.14
Cauliflower	5.60 - 6.63
Celery	5.85 - 6.0
Chickpeas	6.48 - 6.80
Chillies	4.65 - 5.93
Coriander (cilantro)	6.10 - 7.8
Courgette (zucchini)	5.70 - 6.10
Cucumber	5.10 - 5.70
Fennel	5.68 - 6.02
Garlic	5.80
Kale	6.30 - 6.80

Kidney beans	**5.40 - 6.80**
Leeks	**5.50 - 6.17**
Lettuce	**5.98 - 6.13**
Mushrooms	**6.0 - 6.70**
Olives (black)	**6.0 - 7.0**
Olives (green)	3.60 - 4.10
Onions (pickled)	3.70 - 4.60
Onions (red)	5.30 - 4.60
Onions (white)	5.37 - 5.85
Parsnip	5.30 - 5.70
Peas	**5.70 - 6.88**
Peppers (green)	5.20 - 5.93
Peppers (red/bell)	4.80 - 5.20
Pickles	5.10 - 5.40
Potato	**5.90**
Radishes (red)	5.95 - 6.05
Radishes (white)	5.52 - 5.69
Runner beans (string beans)	5.60
Sauerkraut	3.30 - 3.60

Shallots	5.30 - 5.70
Spinach	**6.89 - 7.18**
Sweet potato	**5.30 - 5.60**
Sweetcorn	5.90 - 7.50
Swiss chard	**6.17 - 6.78**
Tofu (soy bean curd)	**7.20**
Tomatoes	3.50 - 4.65
Turnips	5.29 - 6.20
Watercress	**5.88 - 6.03**
Yams	5.50 - 6.81

Notes:

Cucumbers contain cucurbitacin which can cause stomach irritation. For this reason, cucumber is not recommended for those with any kind of stomach complaint. However, I have included it in an upcoming juice recipe, as when used alongside neutral/alkaline ingredients, it's usually far more tolerable than eating alone.

Green cabbage juice is thought to be extremely beneficial for a wide range of digestive disorders including crohn's disease, irritable bowel syndrome and ulcerative colitis. For anyone who hasn't seen the Super Juice Me documentary by Jason Vale, one of the participants tried green cabbage juice daily as part of their stay and had an amazing remission of their symptoms. The documentary is free to watch on YouTube, in case you're interested.

Spinach is one of the most alkaline foods there is, so I recommend always having a fresh bag to hand for your meals, smoothies or juices. I appreciate it's not particularly filling on its own, but its alkaline pH means at least it's going to be safe to eat.

Sweet potatoes come up as mildly acidic/borderline neutral. However, when cooked and served with a handful of spinach I do find them to be GERD friendly. As you heal, you can also try adding a small amount of (reduced fat variety) cream cheese to it. Obviously, if you dollop the cream cheese on thick or opt for a high fat variety, it's not going to be very good for your GERD so be sensible here.

Fruits	Typical pH
Acai	**7.0**
Apples	3.20 - 4.0
Apricot	3.30 - 4.80
Bananas	4.50 - 5.20
Blueberries	3.85 - 4.50
Cherries (black)	3.82 - 3.93
Cherries (red)	3.25 - 3.82
Coconut	**5.50 - 7.80**
Cranberry	2.30 - 2.41
Fig	4.92 - 5.98
Grapefruit	3.0 - 3.75

Grapes	3.50 - 4.50
Jackfruit	4.80 - 6.80
Kiwi	3.10 - 3.96
Lemons	2.0 - 2.60
Limes	2.0 - 2.80
Lychee	4.70 - 5.0
Mango	4.80 - 6.0
Melon	**5.89 - 6.67**
Orange	3.69 - 4.34
Peaches	3.30 - 4.05
Pears	3.50 - 4.60
Pineapple	3.20 - 4.00
Plums	2.80 - 4.30
Pomegranate	2.93 - 3.20
Pumpkin	4.90 - 5.50
Raspberries	3.22 - 3.95
Strawberries	3.00 - 3.90
Watermelon	5.18 - 5.60

Notes:

I appreciate the outlook for fruit is pretty pants, bar the likes of acai, which is incredibly beneficial for GERD and is packed full of antioxidants. Of course, fruit in general is very good for us, but while you're healing from GERD, you're going to need to avoid most fruits, especially citrus fruits. Other fruits (i.e. blueberries) may be acceptable as part of a juice or smoothie, whereby the other ingredients balance the pH out.

Even after you've healed, always try and balance out your juices and smoothies with neutral ingredients (including plenty of vegetables) as high acid fruits can also erode tooth enamel when consumed neat.

Condiments/Miscellaneous	Typical pH
Apple sauce	3.10 - 3.60
Barbecue sauce	4.0
Ketchup	3.90
Mayonnaise	3.60 - 4.0
Mustard	3.50 - 6.0
Pesto sauce	**4.90**
Relish	3.0
Salad cream	3.50 - 3.70
Salsa	4.10
Sour cream	4.40
Tabasco sauce	2.20

Vinegar	2.0 - 3.0

Pesto sauce is a great option for pasta when tomato is out of the question, and it's also great in sandwiches too, especially with chicken and avocado. It does fall on the slightly acidic side, yet for me is an anomaly. Of course, it all depends on how the pesto is made, as some blends will be more neutral than others. If it's store bought and has been sitting on a shelf for days, expect pesto to be more acidic compared with if it was made fresh.

What Do I Mean By 'Alkaline Foods?'

The definition of alkaline is anything above pH 7 in its natural state.

I am not talking about any foods which are considered to 'turn alkaline' once ingested. Because, if they have to pass through your esophagus first, and at a point when their pH is acidic, it will most likely trigger a flare.

The amount of people who have told me that lemons are alkaline is genuinely scary. To me, that's the equivalent of saying lemon juice is good for the back of your retina if you squirt it in your eye, as if it wouldn't sting your eyeball. I think the world has slightly lost its common sense.

I've also had someone tell me alkaline foods turn to 'ash' in the body. Further research leads me to an obscure theory from the 1800s, and all other websites lead to pirate sea shanties. Yeah, sounds proper legit does that.

So please, do not consume any acidic foods that health 'gurus' are saying is 'alkaline eventually', because GERD doesn't work like that and you know it. Once you've healed, it's a different story.

Things That Can Affect Food pH

While the research I have found gives a general estimate of the pH of a food or drink, it's impossible to say with absolute certainty what the pH of any food or drink is, and that's because:

- The variety of the item (i.e. how apples vary in sweetness and therefore pH depending on the variety)
- The growing conditions of the item (i.e. soil quality, plant nutrients, amount of sunlight it received etc.)
- The general condition of the item (i.e. is it underripe, fresh out of the ground or going bad?)
- Whether the item is eaten raw or cooked (cooking can sometimes *slightly* increase the acidity of food, but obviously, do not eat anything raw that is not safe to do so or become afraid to eat cooked foods - use your common sense)
- What is added to the meal when cooking or seasoning, which sometimes can bring the pH of an acidic ingredient down or increase the acidity if the substance added is highly acidic
- Whether the substance has been stored in a liquid (i.e. canned goods)

In addition, if lots of ingredients are added to a meal or a smoothie, the pH level will combine, and depending on the mixture, the pH could increase or decrease. So, if making a meal or a smoothie, you may want to test the pH to check whether the substance as a whole is now more of an acid or alkaline. Depending on what it is you are making, it may be possible to neutralise the entire item (i.e. adding more oat milk to a smoothie).

So, please use the information I have found as an **approximate guide**. Obviously, pH 6.0 and above is preferable, as are foods or drinks that cross the neutral or alkaline threshold above pH 7.0.

As always, you need to **do what feels comfortable for you**. So, if you want to stay ultra alkaline, then that's up to you. I would say so long as you aren't consuming those strong acid foods or beverages (pH 0 - pH 5.0) and you support your stomach with daily probiotics, eating should become more comfortable for you.

Also, consider there may be some anomalies, so if you know of a food or drink to be a general or a personal GERD trigger of yours, always opt for this information over a typical pH reading.

For example, cucumber is excellent in a green smoothie and is incredibly soothing on the skin, yet can have a *slightly* alkaline reading. Likewise, some chilli varieties come up borderline alkaline, as do green peppers, yet we know both to be a general GERD trigger. On the whole though, you should find this list useful.

Note: Some vegetables have alternate names from what they are called in the UK, especially in the USA. So, I have included any differences in terms that I know of in brackets. Failing that, you might have to Google it!

The above list probably has depressed you a little when you realise just how many foods and beverages are acidic, and I'm sorry for that. But at least you know where you might be going wrong now, especially if you drink a lot of cola, coffee, energy drinks or alcohol which can be frightfully acidic.

The easiest way to think about it is to imagine your stomach. If you consume something that has a lower pH than your stomach acid (i.e. it's more acidic than your stomach acid), then it's going to struggle to digest it. The same will also apply if your stomach acid is generally healthy but running low. But by eating foods that are less acidic than your stomach acid, your stomach will have a better chance of being able to break down the food.

Also, I don't expect people to get a strip of litmus paper out every time they eat or drink. Just use your common sense, i.e. if it's not something you'd want to get in your eye, it's probably acidic. But, if you are completely unaware of which foods are acidic, then by all means, do some litmus testing, as you can buy a whole book of test strips for next to nothing.

A final caution is that there is a tonne of pH image charts on Google, all of which have conflicting information. For example, they'll put lime which has a pH of around 2.0 as 'highly alkaline' due to the effect it has on the body in general. Once again for the folks at the back, **I'm talking about the pH of the food or drink in its general state as it enters the esophagus and stomach immediately after swallowing it.** Therefore, for now, it doesn't matter whether a food is healthy or not - the core basis of the decision of what to eat or what not to eat with GERD is whether or not it will burn as you try to digest it or bring on any other symptoms.

3.2 WHAT NOT TO EAT WITH GERD

It's going to come as no surprise that many foods that aren't GERD friendly are in some way acidic due to their pH or simply because they are high in fat. In addition, many cooking or food preparation methods can also make a certain food acidic or generally unhealthy.

I thought it was important to give a specific heading because this is one of the most common questions people ask, in addition to being one of the most important things to know about GERD.

In some cases, the food may have neutral or alkaline pH (aka peppermint), but the ingredient is in some way irritating to the stomach or digestive system. Therefore, **acidity alone is not the only consideration**.

So, as well as any foods which we know to be acidic or a general GERD trigger, some of the main foods specifically that need to be avoided with GERD include:

- Butter
- Cake
- Chilli
- Chocolate
- Cured Meats
- Fried Food
- Ginger

- Lemon
- Mint
- Onions
- Oily foods
- Peppers
- Pineapple
- Processed Foods
- Rich food
- Smoked Foods
- Spicy Food
- Sugar
- Tomatoes

This list isn't exhaustive because there are millions of different food combinations, especially depending on where you live in the world. It's not to say you will directly have a problem with something on the list either.

Also, be aware of whether the food is actually a personal trigger, or whether you ate when you were stressed, already having a flare, too soon before exercise etc. Annoyingly, some foods can trigger me sometimes, and other times they are perfectly fine. Cucumber and cheese are two examples of this. When I have cheese in a sandwich, it can sometimes flare me up. But if I have cheese on a jacket potato, it's perfectly fine.

One theory a subscriber mentioned to me is that heat may have something to do with this, and I think they are right. Hence, melted cheese (Mmmmm!) doesn't cause me an issue. But when I get greedy and slice myself a big chunk and stick it on a cracker, then yes, sometimes I will immediately regret it. Not that you can totally regret eating cheese, though, but you know what I mean. Just pay attention, so you don't keep tripping yourself up.

Foods that relax the LES muscle include:

- Butter or margarine

- Caffeinated beverages
- Chocolate
- Creamy sauces
- Fried food
- High fat meats
- Mayonnaise
- Peppermint
- Salad dressings
- Whole milk dairy products

Foods that stimulate acid production

- Alcohol
- Caffeinated beverages
- Carbonated beverages
- Citrus fruits
- Spicy food
- Tomatoes

Here is a more in-depth explanation of some of the main culprits to help you understand why they are such a hindrance to GERD or even milder bouts of heartburn.

Anything Processed (Especially Fried!)

Imagine a greasy bucket of chicken that's been deep fried. Or any kind of food where you look at the label, and it looks more like a scientific experiment rather than something a human body should digest. These are all foods you should avoid in general, but if you have GERD, they can seriously cause issues. I know these foods taste good, and we all deserve a 'treat', but they aren't doing your body any good, especially your stomach.

The problem is that processed food is highly addictive. Food is also connected to our emotions, so it can be tough to stop eating certain dishes. But, if you genuinely want to recover from GERD, it's not going to happen if you're the sort of person who, when you call up your local takeaway they already know your order. You know?

Nutritious food doesn't have to be boring, nor do you have to 'starve'. If anything, quitting processed food is a time for new discoveries. After all, food is there to fuel our bodies. As I said earlier, would you put the wrong type of petrol (gasoline if you're American) in your car? Then why are we doing this to our bodies? We know if we did that to our car, then it would damage it and most likely would break down too. Our bodies aren't that dissimilar. They too are breaking down because we aren't putting the right things in them. This is your chance to fix this.

All it takes is finding dishes that are healthy and nutritious that you can whip up quickly. Wherever possible, use fresh ingredients. The further away the food is from its original state, the less good it is for you.

For example, a potato versus fries. To turn a potato into fries, it will be cut up, dipped in oil, fried, seasoned with salt etc.

The problem is that processed foods are often the cheapest. Amazingly, you can be obese and have malnutrition at the same time. It's honestly shocking. We need to get back to growing our own food, even if it's just a small window box with some herbs. In the meantime, every effort you can make not to eat that stuff is going to save your health one bite at a time.

It seems so boring to switch to healthy foods and learn about nutrition, I know. Yet, it's often the one thing holding people back the most from getting over all of their problems. Bad skin, weight gain, mood swings and of course GERD - these and so much more can all originate from a poor diet.

Cured Meats

Especially 'smoked' foods such as smoked salmon or smoky

bacon. I think cured meats actually are some of the worst foods when you have GERD because their taste really lingers in your throat.

Rich Foods

Something that really flares me up is rich foods. For example, a cake in a bakery that is oozing with cream, which then makes it ultra high in fat.

Savoury dishes can also be guilty of this too, such as mixing complex flavours that just don't sit well together.

Part of the GERD healing process is stripping down what you eat to involve plain alkaline meals, meaning it's time to ditch rich foods, whether they be fatty, indulgent or too much of an experiment ingredient wise.

Spicy Food

Generally speaking, spicy food is healthy. The problem lies in the acidity of spicy food, with peppers, chillies, herbs, and some spices being particularly bothersome for GERD patients.

In some cultures, spicy food is part and parcel of your daily life. In others, we have competitions about how hot a chilli we can consume. Either way, it's time to dial down on the pH of your food until you feel better.

Ginger

This one might surprise you because ginger is always recommended for any digestive issue. The problem is that ginger contains a lot of heat, and so it can really induce reflux in some people. So, for now, I'd stay clear, especially eating copious amounts, as it can be really overpowering.

Crisps (Potato Chips)

Crisps, as we call them here in the UK, are an easy way to fill a gap but lack any kind of nutrition and can often be high in fat and additives that you really don't want in your body. They are also designed to be eaten in large quantities, making it easy to eat far more than you realise in one sitting.

The crisps that have a coating on them (the orange ones beginning with either D or C if you know the rhyming brand names I'm thinking of) also appear on the list of the unhealthiest foods on the planet, even before you get to what they do for GERD.

If they stain your fingers a luminous shade of orange, what are they doing to your insides?

Healthy Acids

We know that acidic food is bad for GERD, and as I will mention several times throughout this book, this includes healthy acids. Such foods include tomatoes, lemons, chillies, limes, oranges, apricots, strawberries, raspberries and green olives etc.

That doesn't mean these foods aren't healthy in general or that you shouldn't look to reintroduce them into your diet when the time is right.

However, for now, we are working on the pH of these foods at the point at which they are immediately consumed. So no, it doesn't matter if they have an alkalising effect on the body or are super nutritious - they have to pass through your esophagus and stomach first, and if they are going to bring your symptoms on as this happens, **for now, you need to avoid them.** The good news is that this is not going to be forever!

3.3 WHAT NOT TO DRINK WITH GERD

- Alcohol
- Citrus Juices
- Coffee
- Fizzy Drinks (Sodas)
- Hot Chocolate
- Peppermint Tea

Alcohol

Remember my analogy about using an alcohol mouthwash while you have a mouth ulcer? The intensity of the burn is so strong that it makes your eyes water?

Drinking alcohol with any kind of stomach complaint, whether it be GERD or a stomach ulcer, is essentially repeating the exact same process only inside of your body. Only, you can't swill your mouth out with water and apply a topical cream as you can do with a mouth ulcer. Instead, you've created a mini BBQ inside your body, and it's your stomach that's cooking.

For those of you who are social drinkers, suddenly removing alcohol from your routine can cause all sorts of issues. There are probably a lot of people in your circle who won't get it. They might even call you 'boring' for not drinking. Firstly, if that happens, they are not your real friends. Secondly, you have to put yourself first because your GERD cannot heal with the equivalent of lighter fuel being poured on top of it.

On the above mention of mouthwash, you also need to switch to a non-alcohol variety. If you accidentally swallow any, this is really nasty on your stomach in general. However, even the vapours from the alcohol can be enough to trigger a flare-up. So switch to a gentler version.

I appreciate people hate being told not to drink alcohol. But you have to understand I'm coming at this specifically from a GERD perspective, in that if the substance is acidic, it's going to hurt, especially if you haven't recovered yet. In the future, you may need to moderate which drinks you opt for, depending on whether they give you any symptoms or not.

As an example, strong spirits probably aren't going to be your best friend. But, something with a less acidic pH might be something to explore in the future when you're feeling better.

Citrus Juices

There's a reason why they give you orange juice in hotels in the morning to go with your breakfast and not at night before you go to bed. As well as helping you with your digestion and giving you a hefty dose of Vitamin C, stomach acid is more robust in the morning to be able to handle citrus fruits. Hence, if you drink orange juice later in the day, it can ruin your appetite.

Just be aware that although citrus juices are typically very healthy (apart from the sugar content and crap they add to anything that's not freshly squeezed to preserve it), citrus is acidic.

There were times when I would be okay with orange juice, but to be honest, it wouldn't be my first choice if I was having a GERD flare-up. It can also play havoc with your stomach if you drink it in the middle of the day before dinner. So, keep citrus juice to early mornings once you've healed only.

Coffee

I can hear the pit of doom echoing with the screams that fill it. Sorry, I got confused with which genre I was writing in for a second there. It's just, coffee drinkers are extremely attached to their fix. If you didn't already know, coffee is highly acidic. So if you're the kind of person who gulps a cup of coffee and has a cigarette before a stressful work meeting, it's no wonder you're in this situation.

Going cold turkey with coffee or caffeine, in general, is really horrible, and doing so can induce migraines. So you may have to wean yourself off bit by bit if your stomach can handle this.

I'm now personally fine with coffee, though it can be a bladder irritant which isn't much of joy either. When you start to heal and feel ready to reintroduce coffee, make sure you start off by making it as milky as possible. Black coffee is the enemy of GERD, unfortunately.

Lattes are a little less acidic (ask for a 'misto' if you're in the United States, as I've found that you guys actually use espresso in your lattes which is not how we make them in the UK). But, if you're going through a severe flare-up right now, I would try and avoid caffeine wherever possible in favour of water, camomile tea or a green juice (made without ginger, of course).

I'm back to drinking several coffees a day now, if I may gloat. But hey, at least it will be worth it when you can properly enjoy it!

Fizzy Drinks (Sodas)

There's a reason that natural spring water is still and not fizzy. Sodas are bad all round, and as you may notice, it's a bit of a common theme here that all the 'good stuff' basically is too.

The long and short of it is that if your stomach feels hot, painful or uncomfortable, adding in a soda won't shift the feeling. So, for now, give sodas and tonic waters a wide berth.

Hot Chocolate

Thought you could cheat around the 'no chocolate' rule by drinking it instead? Sorry, folks, chocolate is chocolate, whether it's in solid or liquid form. It's also absolutely packed with sugar, which isn't great for reducing inflammation in the body.

Also, the way hot chocolate is served with whipped cream and marshmallows on top also makes it very fatty. As we know, GERD symptoms can be triggered or made much worse by high fat foods and drinks, which is why I do not recommend hot chocolate until you recover.

Peppermint Tea

As illustrated by what happened to me when I went to hospital for advice, having not eaten for two days and in terrible pain with my stomach, drinking peppermint tea with GERD is an absolute no-no. Sadly, a hospital doctor recommended it to me, and it was the utterly wrong advice.

In fairness, peppermint tea is excellent for other digestive issues. But, anything minty with GERD is best avoided until your stomach is in a much better place.

3.4 DITCHING THE SAD DIET

The SAD diet stands for the Standard American Diet and is loathed by dieticians and doctors around the world.

Unsurprisingly considering what we've just covered previously, the SAD diet consists of:

- Butter
- Coffee
- Fried foods
- High fat foods
- Processed food
- Red meat
- Refined grains
- Sugary food and drink

To be honest, it triggered my reflux just typing that out! Now, I'm well aware that not every American eats the SAD diet (hence my love for Californian food), and the SAD diet is also known as the Western Pattern Diet (WPD) because we Europeans have started to adopt this way of eating too. In fact, countries all over the world eat a mixture of foods where some are going to be good for you, and others maybe not so much.

But, what I am saying is that if the above list sounds familiar to you - *regardless* of where you live in the world, then this could be where things have gone wrong. Your body is trying to tell you enough now, especially if your doctor is telling you your GERD is diet related.

Any kind of fatty, processed food is absolutely horrendous for GERD. I don't have an adjective strong enough, to be honest. It hits your stomach, and all the heavy fats just spew out everywhere. Your acid cannot cope, and you get this burning sensation. You might even hiccup a ton and then feel acid in your throat. You need to use the frustration you have as motivation to stop eating this crap and actually heal your body. Even if that means addressing your eating habits with a therapist if it really is that bad. You need to do whatever it takes, and you need to do it now.

If in doubt, remember that the further away food is from its natural state, the worse it will be for you. Why? Because food is supposed to break down as it starts to go bad. So when it has to last on a shelf for weeks on end, manufacturers pump it full of chemicals to stop the decomposition process from happening.

Take the time to look at the ingredients on the packaging. Unfortunately, in America, you guys allow in a lot more chemicals and synthetic ingredients into your food than they do here in Europe. If the ingredients look more like a scientific experiment than a food source, please don't eat it!

Of course, America is a really big place, and every state has its own way of cooking food. I personally spend a lot of time in California, as I mentioned, and the food is the best I have ever tasted anywhere in the world. They have beautiful fresh avocados and healthy smoothies on every corner. In fact, my diet has changed significantly since spending time in California because everything is so healthy and delicious to the point you just don't want to eat crappy food anymore. Yes, it's that good!

I know basic fruits and vegetables seem dull - especially if you prefer processed food - but I promise once you lose your addiction to junk food, you'll feel the best you ever have in your life. Imagine all those vitamins and minerals you are consuming with every bite? Nourishing you from the inside out? I'm sorry, but no amount of fried chicken will do that; in fact, quite the opposite.

Another thing you really want to avoid is too many flavours or ingredients. When you eat out especially, there can be too much going on with your food. With GERD, you want to be keeping your food plain and stripped back. As much as you may want to try more decadent, heavier foods, your stomach simply can't tolerate that right now. This goes for too much seasoning, too - keep the flavours as light and as minimal as possible until you heal. Then you can slowly start to reintroduce new tastes. But in the meantime, you need to go steady.

Portion size can also trip you up. For example, you genuinely wouldn't believe the difference between a typical restaurant portion in the UK versus the USA. That's not me trying to judge; it's just an actual reality that American restaurants tend to give you more food with each serving. In fact, whenever I go to America, I never finish a meal. Instead, I have to ask for a box, so I don't waste any of it.

In some respects, we are starting to catch up with you guys, especially with our pub grub over here in the UK. Even still, I can never believe how much food is brought to the table, even if I just order what I think is going to be a small side dish. Why I'm mentioning portion sizes is that you may not realise just how many calories you're eating because it's standard for you. Given overeating can be a significant GERD trigger, you have to keep this in mind.

There have even been studies that show how certain fast food companies have increased their portions over time. Between the 1960s and 2010s, portions of fries, burgers and soda have increased by as much as 500%. That's impossible to imagine, but basically, where before you'd get a small handful of fries, you now get a giant container of them.

Some restaurants do list nutritional information on the menu. I know it's kind of a buzzkill when they do that, but still, if you're having any kind of digestive issue or are worried about your health in general, you may as well arm yourself with the facts so you can make better choices. It's for your own benefit.

So in many ways, if you do eat the SAD diet in all its forms, you're facing an uphill battle. Such foods are being constantly marketed to you. Those people don't care if the food will give you health problems; they just want to line their pockets.

You may be reading this book from any country, but given the USA has an incredibly high number of GERD sufferers, I think it's really important to address this. I had a quick look at Google Trends, and 'GERD' is also an extremely popular search trend around the world but especially in the USA.

The problem is not only does unhealthy food become addictive, but some people also use it as a source of comfort. Until you make the connection that food isn't just about the taste but how it nourishes your body, you'll be forever stuck in the cycle. If you are depressed, stressed or anxious, you probably don't even care if your food is nourishing you or not. Mental health and food are very closely related. For example, I am a sugar addict. I have used sugar throughout my life to cope with stressful situations. Despite scientists finding that sugar is more difficult to give up than cocaine, I managed to do it, but if I was to have just one little bite of chocolate, I'd soon go back to my old ways. The bad skin and joint inflammation and weight gain would soon follow.

Here's something people don't talk about either, and that's the *pressure* to eat certain foods. Like when I gave up sugar. At work, people would bring in sweet treats, and I'd decline because I was really pleased with how glowy my skin was looking from quitting sugar. Yet, all I'd get in response is, "but it's Christmas, you must eat this, don't be weird." I get it, I do, but then I know if I do eat that treat, I won't just stop there; I'll buy some chocolate on the way home and so on. Listen loud and listen clear: you have to be your own cheerleader here. People aren't always going to understand or support you, but that doesn't matter so long as you stick to it.

So, if you're in America or any other country and you are eating the SAD diet, now is a golden opportunity to change your ways. By doing so, it won't just help your GERD but your overall physical and mental health too. For many of you, it may even extend your life, too, given what we know about the risks associated with many of the foods on the SAD list.

PS: The 'SAD' acronym isn't a coincidence.

3.5 MINDFUL EATING

Mindful eating involves paying attention to *how* you eat food.

Think about this for a second - when was the last time you sat down at a table without any devices and ate a proper meal? These days, most of us eat on the go or in front of a screen. We're all guilty of it, but sometimes not taking the time to notice our food properly can cause digestion issues.

At the very least, a chaotic lifestyle takes your concentration away from the taste of the food. You might even end up eating the wrong or too much food, because you're distracted by whatever you're watching or doing at the time. These distractions mean you may be missing signals about how full you are, or even the suitability of the food you're eating.

It sounds simple enough, but take the time to chew your food properly. When you sit down to eat, try to be free from distractions. A conversation with family or friends around the table is great, because this is proper human interaction. But what you don't want to be doing is guzzling the food down as fast as you can. So, if you're someone who tends to have a rushed breakfast in the morning, or if you don't allow yourself a proper lunch break, you need to redress the balance here.

Also notice your mental state when you try to eat. With GERD in particular, the worst thing you can do is eat when you're stressed or upset. That's because if your body is fired up, it's essentially ready to do battle. All non-essential processes get switched off, and digestion let alone eating more food is going to be difficult, if not impossible if you're not relaxed.

A good analogy here is to liken eating when you are stressed to trying to drive with a nail in your tyre. Sure, the car will move. But will it run at top speed? Will it eventually break down? Can your car function properly when it is dealing with such a critical issue? The nail is in effect, like stress or any other heightened emotional state. Given how the mind and gut are so connected and affected by each other, it makes sense to practice mindful eating.

With GERD, your symptoms may come and go. So how to incorporate mindful eating is to consider how your stomach is feeling before eating any potential triggers, and know when not to push things.

So if you find yourself getting tight in the chest, coughing, the feeling of food getting stuck as you try to eat, or cramps after you eat - you'd benefit from being more aware of yourself, your surroundings and not to mention the type of food you are eating.

No, I'm not saying you have to listen to chanting meditation music when you eat dinner. But at the very least, slow it down. Leave yourself enough time to eat your food, and chew it properly. Take smaller bites rather than six at once. Savour that food and taste the flavour, yes, even if you're eating plain foods because of GERD.

Remember, every day is a clean slate. What can you do differently tomorrow that you didn't do so well today? Could you leave a little extra time to eat your breakfast before rushing out of the door? Think about how you eat food, and see what mindful changes you can make.

So for me when I was at my worst, I'd be trying to eat my sandwich in a newsroom where you could be interrupted with news of a murder at any moment or some other heinous crime. Even overhearing abusive phone calls going on in the background is hardly relaxing. So basically, my body was on 'high alert mode' where digestion is bumped to the back of the queue. I needed to get out of that environment to change things. You may also require adjustments, even if they are less drastic measures like learning to breathe properly.

3.6 WHAT TO DO IF YOU'RE STRUGGLING TO EAT

This is an area where the gastroenterologist I saw for advice and I disagreed massively. According to him, you should still try to eat when you have a GERD flare. Even when it's really bad, and the acid is flying up your throat.

Anytime I tried his method, it was like pouring lighter fuel on a bonfire. So I'm really sorry if any medical professionals disagree with me, but as a patient, my honest feeling is that you should let the acid flare-up subside, even if it's just for a few hours, before challenging the stomach to digest anything.

What I would personally do is just listen to my body. If my stomach felt like a washing machine and was making angry screaming noises (not because it was hungry, but because the acid was way off), then I wouldn't eat. I'd make sure I stayed hydrated but I wouldn't force the food issue.

During an actual flare, my tactic was to drink some camomile tea or a probiotic yoghurt drink as either of these can really help to balance everything out. Plain kefir is also great for this. I wouldn't eat again until the severity of my symptoms settled down, which usually took a couple of hours or if it was late in the evening, the next day.

Sometimes not eating gets difficult, especially if it goes on for a long time. I'm keen to stress that you shouldn't deliberately avoid eating (especially if you feel hungry!). I'm talking about when you *really don't feel hungry* and are in a lot of physical pain with your stomach. When the acid is coming up your throat, you are constantly hiccuping and feel really weak. When you've also seen a doctor to rule out any other conditions too. I do believe the body is being smart here by giving us signals to let us know when to or not to eat - especially when we are ill.

Make sure that when you do eat that it's the right stuff. As I mentioned, my go-to meal was chicken, mashed potatoes, kale and gravy. I must have eaten that about 250 times in a row night after night because I was too afraid to stray off course. Though, it was just the right balance of protein and nutrients. I also took multivitamins and probiotics every day. No, it's not ideal, but when most foods are causing a flare-up, I really think it would do more harm than good to try and force the wrong foods into your diet. You have to wait until you feel better to slowly start introducing them again. As I said, your body is smart, and it will let you know when the right time is to reintroduce acids and broaden your diet once more. It's not going to be forever.

So often, we eat on the go. We're always in a rush. This isn't great for our digestion. While this tip isn't necessarily going to 'cure' GERD, I do think there's something in it. Especially if you're the type of person who eats at their desk while multitasking with several other things. Take the time out to eat your food at a relaxed pace and see if you notice a difference. But the main thing here is to listen to your body, and respond accordingly.

3.7 EATING TOP TIPS

If you have GERD, it's important to eat small meals instead of big ones. Even if the food is really healthy, if there's too much of it going in, your stomach is going to be overfilled. When that happens, out flies the acid.

For some of you, it's going to be a really big adjustment to start having smaller portions. You also might be someone who has to stop learning to eat in response to feeling stressed or bored, which could require seeing a nutritionist or a therapist. But it's something you have to do because with GERD, little and often is the name of the game.

Something I also noticed post-GERD is that my stomach has a bit of a delay in telling my brain it's full. For some people, this can be down to a condition called gastroparesis, which is where the stomach is slow to empty.

I personally think mine is more of a hormonal thing since your hormones control your hunger. The brain releases hormones to let your stomach know you need to eat and when it's full. Sometimes the speed at which that happens can get a little out of sync. Hence people overeat. Anyway, what I do to counteract this is I always stop eating *just before* I get full. I give it a few minutes to see if my stomach catches up. Often this trick saves me from overeating and getting that horrible nausea that follows even from just one extra bite of my dinner.

Eating too close to bedtime or any time in which you will be lying down is also a really bad idea. Again, you're going to have to make some changes here if you normally eat late at night then head to bed. Ideally, you should try to leave a minimum of 3-4 hours between when you last ate and when you go to bed. This is so your stomach has enough time to start digesting the food, rather than gravity working against you.

Also, it's absolutely essential that you don't eat once you've finished your evening meal. For me, this means no eating past 7pm at the latest. Sometimes it can be tempting to have a snack later in the evening, but if you're prone to GERD, this can majorly trigger your symptoms. The only exception would be the consumption of any probiotic drinks or yoghurts.

Another advantage of eating earlier is that you have plenty of time for some camomile tea to soothe your stomach. If you drink copious amounts of liquid before bed, you'll need to get up to pee, so you won't be able to sleep. Your body also won't be able to heal as well because your sleep cycle is constantly disturbed. So, eating earlier has a lot more benefits than it first seems.

When it comes to exercising, you also need to follow the same analogy. We're going to cover what exercises are suitable for GERD in an upcoming chapter. Basically, whatever you do, don't eat a big meal and then go on a treadmill. Or worse still, do yoga or anything else that involves being upside down. It's not that you have to rule out such exercises completely, but you must do them on an empty stomach. Otherwise, it will most certainly trigger you.

I definitely went through a phase where I was scared to eat certain foods because of the memory of how it triggered my symptoms. That's why I made a conscious effort to revisit these foods as soon as I was well enough.

If you think about it, it's totally normal to have such a reaction. You've gone through something massive with your stomach, and it's going to take time to mentally and physically resume normal activity. But you'll get there!

4.0 GERD RECOVERY DIET PLAN

By far, the most requested query I've had for this book is suggestions on what to eat while you are going through GERD. This is totally understandable given your eating is basically the biggest thing that is being affected here.

To be totally honest, if you are expecting a really vast diet plan with tons of recipes, you are going to be disappointed because if I did that when your stomach is in a state of extreme pain and imbalance, it's going to cause you more harm than good. Instead, my mantra for GERD diets is to follow everything we've just covered, i.e. small but nutritious meals that are simple in nature without trying to overload you.

This is exactly what I followed when I was trying to recover from GERD because I found every time I did stray off course, it would flare my symptoms up.

For me, telling you about the foods that have helped me as a former GERD sufferer is based on quality rather than quantity. There's no point writing endless amounts of recipes, especially if I include foods that I didn't personally eat or that I know won't help you. It's also going to be unrealistic to eat lots of different food types until you feel ready to. So let's stick to what's actually going to help you until you reach the point where you feel well enough to start reintroducing more foods.

Before I utter a word of advice on how I healed my GERD, let me be clear that even if your diet is amazing, the changes are going to take a while to kick in. That's not because my method doesn't work; it's because, being completely realistic, the body takes time to heal, yes, even when you are doing all the right things! Also, if you fix your diet but continue to be chronically stressed, you may as well not even bother. So, you have to really line up all your ducks in a row here, and I really do mean all of them.

Before you rule a food out as a 'trigger', I also want you to consider if anything else could have caused the reaction. For example, were you already in the middle of a flare-up, or were you stressed when you ate whatever it was?

Even if you aren't a fan of my recipes (it pays to be realistic here, we all have different tastes), then the key is to keep your food as plain as possible. I know, I'm really sorry that it may mean your food is bland. Remember, it's not going to be forever. For the most part, you will be able to return to eating most foods, bar anything in the SAD/WPD diet (especially fried/greasy foods).

Another thing to remember is that the 'flavour' of foods is often artificial. Processed foods are pumped with so much sugar and additives that they actually become addictive. Our body doesn't even know what to do with most of it because it's essentially alien. So what I'm saying is, those 'amazing' tastes aren't as good as you think.

Once again, there is a mismatch between what nature intended we eat and what we actually eat. So, it's no wonder GERD and many other conditions are so common. Instead, we're going to get back to basics in the most GERD friendly way possible.

The purpose of eating is not to help you destress or fill an emotional hole - it's to gain the energy and nutrients that your body needs. Unless you realign this core purpose, you're most likely going to continue to have issues with GERD or other health related problems.

Note: Consult a doctor before making any changes to your diet if you have any food intolerances or any other serious medical conditions beyond GERD.

GERD Friendly Food List

- Acai
- Almond milk
- Artichokes
- Avocado
- Broccoli
- Brown rice
- Brussels sprouts
- Cabbage (green)
- Cabbage (white)
- Camomile tea
- Carrots
- Cauliflower
- Celery
- Chicken (breast)
- Chickpeas
- Coconut
- Coriander (cilantro)
- Courgette (zucchini)
- Gluten free bread
- High fibre + low sugar cereals
- Kale
- Kefir
- Kidney beans
- Leeks
- Lettuce
- Melon
- Mushrooms

- Oat milk
- Oats
- Olives (black)
- Peas
- Pesto
- Potato
- Spinach
- Sweet potato
- Sweetcorn
- Swiss chard
- Tofu
- Water
- Watercress
- Wholemeal bread/wraps
- White rice
- Yams

The GERD friendly food and drink ingredient list isn't huge, but it should give you something to go off when trying to plan meals, or if you're out in a restaurant and are stuck for what to order.

Try to keep the number of ingredients and the seasoning you add to any dish to a minimum. Once you start to overcomplicate food on a delicate stomach, trouble often follows.

The Alkaline Diet

Most of the content that's about to follow in section 4.1 and beyond is related to eating alkaline. Basically, the reasoning behind this is that while you recover, alkaline food and drink are going to stress the stomach the least because we're keeping the pH at a safe level, unlike when you consume highly acidic foods.

But by the same token, I'm also not suggesting that we are trying to 'turn the body alkaline' or any of these extreme claims.

Instead, I'm simply thinking of the esophagus and the stomach in a fragile state. Therefore, with alkaline foods, the aim is to have the food pass through these regions as comfortably as possible without inflicting further irritation.

I want to clear this up just because the whole alkaline diet movement can get quite intense, as I mentioned with some people claiming foods 'turn to ash' inside you. I mean, I know your stomach burns and all, but that doesn't mean it's literally cremating your food!

So please keep the whole pH thing in perspective here because, as I have said, at some point, you'll want to introduce acidic foods again, especially the healthy acids that are packed full of nutrients. It's just not something to do for now so that you have a chance to recover.

A Problem I Have With The Majority Of GERD Cookbooks

I'm sure they mean well, but looking at some of the recipes in these GERD cookbooks, I have a strong suspicion the author has never experienced GERD themselves.

That's not to say they are bad full stop or that you won't enjoy them at some stage, or even that the recipes are definitely going to cause you a flare-up. However, going on the basic principles of alkaline foods, grilling over frying, nutrition first and eating small portions - if that's not what the recipe instructs, it may cause you a problem.

I'll give you some examples of recipes that make me shriek:

'Maple BBQ Salmon' - Barbeque honey has a pH of 4.0, which makes it acidic, and barbeque, similar to cured or smoked meats, can be very troublesome for GERD. Even salmon or other super 'fishy' meats, as healthy as they may be, have a strong taste to them and may encourage some of the unpleasant side effects, such as when certain foods can repeat on you.

'Apricot Chicken Thighs' - Apricot is also acidic, so yes, while it may be healthy for you, as we've already established, even healthy acids need to be cut from your diet until you heal from GERD. I also have an issue with the mixing of chicken and apricot because you're mixing flavours that don't particularly go well together, and this in itself can cause GERD. Also, chicken thighs have a high fat content, especially with the skin left on. Instead, chicken breast is much leaner.

'Cheesy Broccoli Loaded Bakes' - The idea of eating anything 'loaded' or oozing with cheese when you have GERD is nauseating. The fat content is simply too high, and it will induce a flare, which could set you back a few days. It's also missing a golden opportunity to get some much needed nutrition in you. Sure, cheese and broccoli are nutritious in many ways, but not when it's delivered in such an indulgent fatty way. Save such treats for when you can handle them again, so you know they will actually be a treat and not a fire breathing exercise.

'Veggie Quesadillas' - Well, this one website - a top-ranking result for 'GERD friendly recipes' is turning more into a comedy show now. The recipe calls for jalapenos, salsa, chipotle chilli powder, refried beans, peppers and onions. At a push, you could tailor this recipe to use alkaline veggies and ditch the sauces and creams. But, you know full well some poor suspecting folk are going to make this recipe as is and be in agony.

In summary, there are a lot of irresponsible people making GERD cookbooks simply with profit in mind and not the people who are actually desperate for foods that won't make them feel worse. So please be careful out there!

Onto some GERD friendly food ideas written by an actual recovered patient. Be prepared to spot the difference.

4.1 BREAKFAST

Do you leave yourself enough time to eat breakfast in the morning? If not, this will need to change so that you not only have time to eat properly but are relaxed when you do so, even if you only have five or ten minutes. If you can pop some headphones on and listen to some relaxing spa music while you eat, instead of scrolling through the news and depressing yourself about the state of the world from the moment you wake up - this is even better.

Ideally, I'd encourage everyone to develop a morning stretching routine before they eat breakfast so that all of your muscles are gently warmed up to face the day ahead. It also means you're not going straight from lying down to eating, as there's a bit of a transition alongside showering and getting ready for the day.

Any one of the following options I would personally recommend for GERD because the pH is going to be stomach acid friendly and give you nutrients and energy at the same time.

If you have a flare upon waking, stick to alkaline liquids and try to eat at lunch instead - you should regain your appetite 2-3 hours after the consumption of any greens or probiotics in particular.

Avocado Toast

- Wholemeal seeded bread
- Avocado

Toast is amazing when your stomach is off, but especially with GERD. I recommend wholemeal bread as it's classed as a complex carb. With white bread, all of the good stuff has been stripped out. But with wholemeal (especially super seeded varieties), it's all left in, and it will keep you fuller for longer.

If you're having severe symptoms, you may want to try dry toast first and slowly reintroduce a small quantity of butter when you feel better. If you lather butter on thick, you're going to be in trouble. So instead, use your knife to carve only a thin slither of the butter and distribute it across the full piece of toast.

Alternatively, if you're not quite ready to reintroduce butter back into your diet, my favourite restaurant in Pasadena (Urth Caffé) notes they use olive oil on their avocado toast. They also top theirs with ripe Hass avocados, almond cheese and micro cilantro (coriander to any fellow Brits reading).

Acai Bowl

- Acai powder or frozen acai pulp
- 2 Bananas
- Almond milk or plain yoghurt
- A handful of spinach (optional)
- Mango (optional)
- Frozen berries (optional)
- Avocado (optional)
- Granola/seeds/nuts (toppings)

Don't be fooled by the name, as acai is actually alkaline! Just don't ask me to help you pronounce it. (Ah-sigh-ee).

I made quite a late discovery of acai, and further research has informed me that not only is it incredibly dense in antioxidants, but it's thought that acai may also help to protect and repair the lower esophagus after it has been damaged by GERD.

Acai can be purchased in many different formats and is delicious as a frozen treat too. However, the easiest way to find acai is through powder form, as you can add it to a blender to make an acai bowl. Or you can find frozen acai pulp, and if using a frozen variety, make sure it's pure acai with no added sugars or other nasties you don't need.

If you're at the start of your GERD recovery journey, you can simply blend the acai with plain yoghurt or oat milk. Adding in a banana or avocado will give it some bulk.

For everyone else, grab your blender and add a sachet of frozen acai pulp. You'll need to break it up into a few chunks first, and you may also want to soften it under a warm tap or leave it in the fridge for a few hours to defrost so that it's not rock solid.

Add your banana to the blender. Now, if you're already into the healing stage of your GERD, you could swap the banana out for mango. Though as mango is mildly acidic, don't add it if you're at the start of your journey. Likewise, this recipe has an option of adding berries such as blueberries, blackberries or strawberries - the same applies as to whether you are up to this or not. Don't worry if you're not, because the main thing is going to be the acai. But the ability to customise the recipe as you feel better also means it will keep things interesting in the long term.

Also, if you have any leftover spinach hanging around, you can also throw a handful in the blender too. I mention this because sometimes it can be difficult to use the whole bag up, though this step isn't necessary. Avocados can also enhance the texture of the bowl, but it is up to you whether you add it or not, as the banana will help thicken it up too.

Add in your oat milk or yoghurt. Now, I know in America you guys use the word 'cups', but to us Brits, a cup is what we drink tea out of. So instead, fill up the blender with the almond milk so that you'll get enough to get a thick consistency, but not so thick it will stick to the blender, which is around 200ml (7 fl oz) of milk.

Blend the mixture for around 30-40 seconds, so it is one solid blend. If it's too runny, add in a banana or some avocado to thicken it back up. If it's too thick, add some more almond milk or even a small drop of water just to get some liquid in there. It should feel slightly thicker than a smoothie. Once you're happy with the consistency, pour it into a bowl.

You can then add any toppings you see fit. Granola or even oats can add a particularly nice crunch. Grab your other banana, slice it into thin slithers and arrange it nicely on top. If you're feeling up to it, add a handful of berries or even some nuts such as almonds. Work to your personal tastes and preferences along with what you can currently handle.

Green smoothies or juices

For those who can't face eating or want to consume their energy on the go, then a green smoothie or juice is going to be your best pal. Quite simply, most greens are not only alkaline but full of nutrition.

Don't hate me, but you'll need a blender and a juicer for this recipe. But, the good news is that if you have a couple of smoothie cups, you'll normally get enough for two days. If you still can't be arsed, then skip the avocado and juice the rest of the ingredients.

Note: We have some *mildly acidic* ingredients in this one, but avocado, carrots, celery and spinach to help balance the pH. Remove any ingredients as you see fit - it's more important the recipe is comfortable for you than anything else.

1x avocado (1 small one or half a large one)

4 x celery sticks
2 x carrots
1 x apple
1 x pear
½ a cucumber
Generous handful of spinach

Wash all the ingredients and drain in a colander. Juice the celery, carrots, apple and pear. Chop the avocado and cucumber and add into the blender. Add in your juice and blitz in the blender for another ten seconds until smooth. Transfer into a smoothie cup with a lid and drink up.

If you've made enough for two cups, keep the other cup refrigerated. You may also wish to add some ice into the blender when you transfer everything if you live in a warm climate, which will keep the ingredients fresher for longer.

All of these ingredients will keep your essential minerals and vitamins topped up. Celery, in particular, is great for our stomach acid. Now, some suggest juicing celery on its own and that there's 'no benefit in adding it with other ingredients' - I personally don't agree with this because eating celery has gotten to be better than not doing so at all. Plus, celery juice has an acquired taste. If you're not used to juicing, it's a bit of a baptism of fire taste wise if it's not mixed with other ingredients.

So, don't get too precious about it, just get those greens in you! As a general guide, here are some fruits and veggies that are either best put through a juicer or a blender.

Essentially, if the item has a high water content, then it's great for juicing, though something such as an avocado or banana won't give you much liquid and in fact, needs more liquid to be added to the blender, so it doesn't go too thick. There are also some crossovers, such as spinach, that work great in either.

I'm not going to list things like oranges or strawberries for now, as I want you to keep the acid content down while you heal. But, you should explore as much of a rainbow diet as possible, as well as which foods work better in a juicer or a blender as soon as you start to feel better.

Great for juicing:

- Apples
- Beetroot
- Carrots
- Celery
- Spinach

Great for blending:

- Acai
- Avocados
- Bananas
- Blueberries
- Kefir
- Plant-based milk (i.e. oat or almond)
- Spinach

Top tip: Have a look at some of the amazing smoothie powders that can be added to your smoothie, especially green or antioxidant powders. In some cases, it can make it much easier to use these versus fresh ingredients or as an added boost to really cover all bases.

Fibre Rich Cereals

Fibre heavy cereals accompanied with plant-based milk are another option you can try. I throw out caution here as most cereals are full of crap (your breakfast isn't supposed to look like a rainbow or a chocolate lake), and disturbingly these types of cereals are mostly aimed at children.

Instead, I'm talking about cereals that have a much more healthy edge and are low in sugar while high in fibre. So, check out your local supermarket or health food store to explore the full range of options available.

I've actually noticed some of the big breakfast cereal companies are now making high fibre cereals with added prebiotics or probiotics, which is fantastic.

Kefir Drink

Kefir is a relatively new discovery for me and is actually something I tried after a bout of jet lag when my stomach had no idea what time of day it was.

Kefir is a type of yoghurt drink that is made from fermented milk. Now, provided you don't have any intolerances to the ingredients, and you opt for a plain flavour rather than anything full of sugar, you should notice it gives you a soothing effect that makes it easier to eat your lunch later.

Obviously, read the ingredients before drinking kefir and monitor how you feel after taking it. If you're all good, there's no reason why you can't continue as an alternative to a heavier breakfast or as a healthy snack. Given how plain it is, the drink shouldn't cause an issue as your stomach tries to break it down, especially in comparison to fried breakfast options.

Porridge (Oatmeal)

When it comes to porridge (or oatmeal as you call it in the USA), you'll struggle to find a better GERD friendly breakfast option that's slow releasing, nutritious and cost-effective. With so many different ways to serve it up, there's no reason why you can't find a recipe that suits you.

I personally buy a large bag of porridge oats from a budget

supermarket. One bag will feed me for about three months, working out as something as ridiculous as 2p (2.5 cents) per serving.

I usually make it with water, but you can try a delicious plant-based milk such as oat or even coconut. Making it with regular milk is also fine if you're okay with dairy, but I'd opt for a low fat option to be on the safe side.

I add in some chia seeds on the top for protein. The benefits of chia seeds include:

- Contains fibre, protein, calcium, manganese, magnesium, phosphorus, zinc and B Vitamins
- Antioxidant properties
- Can aid weight loss
- High in omega-3 fatty acids (the good kind of fat!)
- Can help reduce blood pressure
- Can help reduce inflammation
- Easy to incorporate into your diet
- Not expensive (the ones I buy cost £1/$1.30 USD a pack)

Honestly, there are so many different seeds that will add even more flavour to a bowl. Some people also like to top porridge off with honey or berries, but go with what you like and what your stomach is saying.

If you are going to add some honey on top, don't add the nasty cheap stuff that's full of sugar. Manuka honey has a grading system known as UMF (Unique Manuka Factor) - the higher the UMF score, the better. The top quality honey can get expensive, so this really is an optional step, but it's known to have incredible healing properties.

4.2 LUNCH

Lunch can be an awkward meal of the day with GERD because if you've had a really stressful morning, you might not feel like eating.

So assuming you do have at least some appetite, you should once again proceed with a light, healthy bite. But, don't force the situation if you can't eat. Or just opt for something small with a view to addressing any stressors that could be affecting your eating habits.

As with all of your meals, it's also good to try to establish a regular window to eat lunch in. So, for example, if you eat lunch at 12pm one day, try and eat at a similar time the next day rather than waiting until 2pm. The obvious exception being if you're having a flare and need to wait a while until you eat again.

You can also take a probiotic tablet before eating lunch or try a probiotic drink or probiotic yoghurt after eating lunch.

Avoid the temptation to eat fast food or even a really heavy lunch so that you don't mess up how hungry you are for dinner in the evening.

Alkaline Soups

- Vegetable stock
- Bone broth (optional vegetable stock replacement)
- Any alkaline vegetables of your choice
- Light seasoning (i.e. salt and pepper to taste)

Alkaline soups are an excellent choice for lunch. You have the option here of purchasing a fresh soup, a soup cleanse from a health company or making some soup yourself. Just avoid super processed soups that have been sitting on the shelves for months, as the nutritional content will not be as good.

In particular, the heavy liquid content of soups and broths makes them ideal for a variety of ailments. I mention the term 'alkaline' as you want to be avoiding tomatoes or anything with heavy seasoning or flavours. Likewise, avoid adding high fat cuts of meat into your soup, such as beef.

Though interestingly, some sources swear by bone broth as it is rich in gelatin and cartilage, which can help to restore the damaged esophagus, as well as being abundant in minerals and electrolytes. From what I've found, bone broth appears to be much lower in fat than beef also.

Some of the other ingredients to base your soup around could include sweet potato, potato, carrot, celery, chicken, cabbage, leeks or spinach.

You can basically cook any of these, add them into a blender along with your vegetable stock and some cornflour for thickening and then place them back in the pan to finish off.

Gently heat your blend in a warm pan, and season with a pinch of salt and pepper to ensure the flavour is balanced while ensuring the soup remains GERD friendly. Making any kind of soup shouldn't feel complicated or time consuming - just get the blended ingredients in a pan and play around until the taste hits the spot.

For any winning formulas, why not batch cook the soup next time and freeze it so that you'll always have some on hand if you need it?

I do recommend serving the soup with a wholemeal bread roll, just so it adds some interest to the meal and helps to fill you up. Again, don't add lashings of butter to the bread roll; otherwise, you'll undo all your hard work!

Chicken Sandwich

- Wholemeal bread
- Low fat butter or vegetable spread
- Cooked chicken breast strips (or vegan chicken alternative)
- Avocado
- Spinach leaves
- Pesto (optional extra)

Chicken is on my dinner menu, so it's not something I necessarily recommend eating several times a day. But, if you're not planning on having chicken for dinner, then it can make for a GERD friendly lunch idea.

I would always advocate making a chicken sandwich with wholemeal bread, preferably seeded. Though, you could always try a roll or wrap to spice things up (it's about as much 'spice' as you're allowed with GERD, one jests).

If you are having a fairly okay day, then lightly buttering the bread is fine, as we discussed with the toast. If you're not, then either use a low fat spread, vegetable spread or try spreading some avocado across the bread so it's not dry. In general, chicken, avocado and spinach work great together in a sandwich.

There's also a well known retailer here in the UK that makes a chicken and avocado sandwich with Parmigiano Reggiano cheese mayonnaise that I also find to be GERD friendly.

Don't smother your sandwich in heavy condiments or anything ultra fatty or processed, please.

Tomatoless Salad

- Mixed bag of salad leaves (200g)
- ½ avocado (sliced)
- Olive oil
- Small handful of chopped chives

I appreciate the word 'salad' often generates a collective sigh. But, we need a GERD friendly lunch option for vegans as well as those trying to lose weight. Plus, there are plenty of ways you can tailor your salad to your preference taste wise.

With the above recipe, you're going to put four teaspoons of olive oil into a jar along with the chives and shake - this will be the seasoning that you add to the salad leaves in a bowl or container. Add in the sliced avocado last and mix it all up. It really is that simple. Obviously, if you find there's too much there, then save some for later, as you can add the salad with whatever you make for dinner.

Really, the only thing you need to avoid with this simple salad or any other salad recipe is tomato or acidic dressings such as lemon, balsamic vinegar or mustard. Keep it lean and green, and you're good to go!

Sweet Potato

- Sweet potato
- Spinach
- Low fat butter or low fat cream cheese (optional)

Sweet potatoes are packed full of nutrients and are generally very gentle on the stomach. You can either eat sweet potatoes as an alternative to a regular jacket potato or cut the sweet potato up as a healthier option than fries.

Assuming you'll be baking your sweet potato, you'll need to give it a good wash first. Poke holes in the potato and place it on a lined baking tray. It will need around an hour in the oven at 220ºC (200ºC fan), at which point it should be soft and tender.

Obviously, this option is for when you have a little more time to kill or if you work at home, so you're able to let it cook through for a while.

Now, you may want to add a small amount of butter or low fat cream cheese, though you may need to skip these if you're going through a flare. Eating it without a topping will give you some nutrients and may be the only option if you're really struggling right now. But, as you progress, you'll be able to start enjoying some more flavourful toppings, so long as you don't go too high fat. This is why I always state any toppings are 'optional'.

4.3 DINNER

When I was going through the worst of my GERD struggles, I ate the same dinner night after night for months on end, and this is the same dinner I talked about in my YouTube video.

The reason this dinner worked for me was that it was gentle on my stomach. You'll notice none of the ingredients and especially the way they are prepared add any harsh acids. I also did not eat large portions of this meal, sticking to only what I needed before I felt full.

Chicken, Mashed Potato, Kale And Gravy

- 2 chicken breasts
- 2 large potatoes
- 1 pack kale
- 1 beef stock cube
- 1 tablespoon cornflour

Heat the oven to gas mark 6 (200 C/400 F).

Peel and chop potatoes into quarters and place in a steamer/pan to boil.

Add the cornflour into a mug and slowly add just enough water to make a smooth paste. Put the stock cube into a different mug and add boiling water. Stir until dissolved.

Add the stock to the cornflour mixture and stir.

Place the chicken breasts in a small ovenproof dish and pour some of the gravy mixture onto the chicken to add taste. Cook the chicken for 25-30 minutes, turning halfway through.

Add the kale in the steamer or another pan and cook for about 15 mins.

Take the chicken out of the oven, then mash the potatoes.

Drain the kale. Place the chicken, mashed potatoes and kale on a plate and spoon over the rest of the gravy.

The above recipe was written by my mother, who cooked me this meal hundreds of times over because for so long, it was all I could manage for dinner. It's incredibly plain to eat, not least because the chicken and mashed potato isn't seasoned. Instead, the gravy would provide some light flavour. This dish also gives a good mix of nutrients without being in any way overwhelming.

If you want to change up the stock cube flavour, that's up to you, as it might seem strange to mix chicken and beef but for this particular dish it works well. Also, because it's just a stock cube and not a fatty cut of actual beef, it's also safe to eat with GERD.

Gravy can be acidic, but this is usually when acidic meat juices are added. With stock cubes and without heavy seasonings etc, it's going to have a gentler pH. I was personally fine even when I was at my worst with this particular gravy recipe.

For any vegans or vegetarians reading, I now mostly eat plant-based foods. There are plenty of dupe chicken substances you can try. Alternatively, use your favourite plant-based protein that isn't acidic and will go well with kale, mash potato and gravy.

Warning: As dull as this meal may seem to eat each night for dinner, only proceed onto my other dinner recipe suggestions or any other GERD friendly meals when you start to notice an improvement in your symptoms. That's because, from personal experience I found that the last meal of the day can have the biggest impact on how you sleep and how you feel when you wake up. You don't have time to burn off the food throughout the rest of the day if you overeat, and you have less time to settle your stomach with camomile tea, probiotic milk or kefir. So, stick with it until all your other changes are starting to take impact (i.e. less stress, probiotics etc). You'll know when you feel ready, and most importantly I want you to start to enjoy every bite again, not end up back at square one.

Wholewheat Wraps

- Wholewheat wraps
- Roast chicken pieces or vegan sausage
- Avocado
- Lettuce/salad leaves
- Rocket (arugula)
- Shredded lettuce

A bit of a basic one where wraps are concerned, seen as we can't go crazy with tomatoes, peppers, cheeses, sauces etc. However, this is a recipe that's easy to throw together and is great for warmer weather when you might not feel like gravy and mash potatoes.

If purchasing cooked roast chicken, warm it through on the grill. Alternatively, follow the cooking instructions for the vegan sausages, which will need to be baked in the oven.

Grab your wholemeal wrap and also give it a warm through in the oven. Chop up the protein you've chosen and add it into the wrap.

Add some small cubes of avocado, along with lettuce or salad leaves. Rocket can also help fill up the wrap with plenty of alkaline greens.

If you're feeling particularly hungry, you can serve the wraps with some kale salad or sweet potato cubes.

Tempeh Burger

This one isn't a 'how to make it' as I actually have had this in a plant-based restaurant and wanted to recommend it to you.

Basically, the burger can be bought off the shelf or homemade and contains tempeh, lentils and nuts. The burger is grilled rather than fried, and can be topped with something such as pesto, avocado and lettuce. The bun is also wholewheat.

As a side dish, you can try a kale salad or sweet potato hash as with the last recipe. If you want to use a regular potato, you can make healthy fries by grilling rather than frying them and adding seasoning to taste.

So essentially, it's a burger that isn't fried, nor is it served with onions, ketchup or anything remotely greasy. This means it looks and tastes like a treat, but doesn't contain any of the usual culprits.

I have to say that in general, plant-based food, particularly 'meat' substitutes are very agreeable in a GERD sense.

Now, you might be reading this wanting more recipes. But, you have to remember this is my healing story as a GERD patient. As I mentioned, I ate this same meal every night for dinner until I felt well enough to start introducing new foods. That's because we are starting with a small rotation of foods we trust and gradually building outwards as we feel stronger, rather than trying to overload our system when it's currently in disarray.

If you are at the stage where you've tried these meals and you're getting bored, there are some other things you can do, and that is to factor in any foods you've been able to eat up to now to make a meal from those. If you are still struggling to eat barely anything, then I'd recommend you probably aren't ready to expand into eating new foods, and you need a few more weeks of simple alkaline foods and probiotics.

In addition, some of the options I mentioned for lunch could also be tried as dinner options. For example, a sweet potato and a side salad.

Know you're definitely better and ready to move onto more foods? Recap my GERD friendly foods list at the start of this chapter.

4.4 SNACKS

With GERD, you might not feel like a snack, and I definitely wouldn't advise any after eating your main meal at night, in case you overeat by accident.

However, if your stomach is still in pain and you're afraid to eat a bigger meal, or if you're looking to fill a gap then there are plenty of GERD friendly snacks. Just be sure to only eat a small amount of snacks so that you don't mess up your appetite.

It's probably not going to be much of a shock that the likes of potato chips, sausage rolls, chocolate or any other kind of nasty processed food is not going to be on the list. That's because with every bite, we need to get you closer to a recovery rather than further away from it.

Almonds

Nuts contain healthy fats that we need along with nutrients and vitamins that are good for everything from our brains to our skin. Almonds are certainly a GERD friendly snack, as they can help ward off pangs of hunger when it's not convenient to eat, and because they aren't acidic, they won't give any ill effects after you swallow them.

Almonds are also great for adding a crunch to your oatmeal or even your smoothies if you don't like eating them whole. Try a small handful in between breakfast and lunch and see how you get on.

Boiled Eggs

In general, dairy products aren't recommended for GERD. However, boiled eggs have a typical pH of 7.6, and can be as alkaline as 9.2. Eggs are also delicious when slightly runny, and are perfect with some wholemeal toast.

Coconut Chips

Many snack companies make dried coconut crisps/chips. Essentially, think potato chips only made from dried coconut with no frying, additives, or even added ingredients. The coconut is gently baked at a low temperature, where it develops a satisfying crunch. Although coconut chips aren't super filling, they are a much healthier alternative than most things you'll find down the snack aisle of any store.

Edamame Beans

Another ultra healthy treat is edamame beans. They are actually far more delicious than they look for anyone who hasn't tried them before! Edamame beans are also free from cholesterol, low in saturated fat and high in fibre.

Peanut Butter Apple Slices

Leave this snack as an indulgent treat, as it's not quite as healthy as the others! Peanut butter helps to balance the acidity of a slice of an apple, and the two flavours go great together. Always look for a high quality peanut butter, and watch out for the sugar and fat content.

Probiotic Yoghurts

We're going to be covering probiotics in great detail shortly, but it's worth mentioning that probiotic yoghurts also make for an excellent GERD friendly snack and can even soothe some of the symptoms you are experiencing.

As a general rule, try to avoid fruit flavours that are highly acidic or anything too berry heavy, as even though yoghurt is fairly neutral, some fruits are going to be more gentle than others.

4.5 ADDITIONAL SUPPLEMENTS

I know you might be struggling to eat right now, but if there's one thing you should be taking alongside probiotics, then it's a multivitamin. Stating the obvious, a multivitamin isn't a replacement for eating a healthy diet, but there are two ways in which it can help the situation. Firstly, if you are struggling to eat, you may become depleted in certain nutrients, so I always think it's a good idea to keep topped up (especially with things such as Vitamin C/D).

The other important point is that magnesium, which is found in most vitamin supplements, can be incredibly beneficial to GERD sufferers. Magnesium is thought to reduce spasms of the lower esophageal sphincter, which prevents the release of acid into the esophagus. In some cases, magnesium deficiency can also be an indicator of low stomach acid. So, what that means is that some patients actually develop GERD because they don't consume or absorb enough magnesium. So, ensure you are getting your daily recommended allowance of magnesium alongside all other key vitamins.

Foods which naturally contain magnesium include green leafy vegetables (such as spinach and kale), as well as nuts, bananas, figs and raspberries, to name but a few examples. While you should, of course, look to get your nutrients from your food, when your health is a little off I do think a multivitamin containing magnesium can be helpful too.

No, taking a multivitamin on its own is not going to cure you. But that doesn't mean it's not worth it. Instead, it's one of the many little steps on your walk, which is going to take you from feeling like utter crap with GERD, to eventually being able to eat without having to second guess yourself.

Turmeric

This is a cautionary suggestion, as unfortunately, GERD sufferers either find turmeric to be amazing or a trigger. But, because turmeric is so widely praised for its anti-inflammatory properties, it's well worth a mention.

Turmeric has a typical pH of between 7.4 and 9.2 making it highly alkaline. It has a wide range of health benefits. To release the inflammation busting properties of turmeric, it must be combined with black pepper.

One idea is to make yourself a fresh soup and add turmeric and black pepper to it. Soups may be helpful for a lot of you because you can control the pH, especially if you make it yourself and avoid any acidic ingredients.

Obviously, take it easy and monitor your symptoms. Also, consider starting tumeric when you are starting to slightly feel better, rather than trying to overload yourself with too many supplements when you are at your worst.

What I certainly don't want is anyone thinking they 'have' to consume every single type of supplement or recommendation, especially when they are struggling. If you find turmeric doesn't agree with you, move on for now and come back to it in a few weeks when you feel ready.

4.6 CAMOMILE TEA

Camomile tea basically kept me sane throughout my GERD struggles. I should point out that camomile has two spellings, including 'chamomile'. Neither is strictly incorrect; it's more of a stylistic preference depending on where you are based. In the UK, we tend to use the Middle English spelling of 'camomile'. But, you may find companies spelling camomile tea as 'chamomile tea', which is perfectly okay.

Camomile tea in itself is not going to 'heal you'. However, it's absolutely brilliant at taking the edge off your symptoms, especially with any kind of stomach related problem. Furthermore, camomile is caffeine-free and has tranquilising properties, meaning if you are stressed, and this is flaring up your GERD, it couldn't be a better thing to consume.

I personally recommend drinking camomile after every meal, especially if you are experiencing a flare. In particular, I used to find drinking a cup of camomile after my evening meal at night would really keep my symptoms at bay before I went to sleep.

I have only had one single person comment on my video that camomile tea didn't work for them out of thousands who said it helped soothe their symptoms. There is always one!

The quality of camomile tea is going to differ depending on the brand you purchase. Please obtain from buying any weird flavour combinations that probably won't agree with your stomach. Keep it to simply 'camomile tea'.

If it's a colour other than deep yellow, fizzy, contains caffeine or has been sitting on the shelf for days in liquid form - it's not camomile tea.

How To Make Camomile Tea

I don't think I've ever felt more British than writing about how to make tea. There is an art to making all types of tea which will affect the flavour and overall drinking experience.

With camomile tea, it's absolutely essential you don't scold it. Remember, it's made from flowers, after all. Instead, you want to use 80°c/176°F water. Luckily, we have a fancy kettle my brother gave us, which has a '80°c' button. For everyone else, you want to cut the heat before the kettle boils or before you start to see too many bubbles of boiling water on the stove.

You could also use a thermometer to check the water temperature if my less than scientific explanation didn't cut it for you, which I highly suspect is the case. Place the camomile tea bag into a cup and pour the water in.

Give it a couple of minutes before you drink it so that the camomile has had enough time to infuse into the water.

If using a loose camomile tea variety, you'll need a specialist teapot or mug that filters out the flowers when you pour the tea into your mug.

Loose vs Pressed Camomile Tea

It's also possible to find loose camomile that needs to be steeped for 3-5 minutes before you drink it. Also, some tea bags (usually pyramid shaped) can contain loose camomile.

The other alternative is pressed camomile, which is most commonly found within standard teabags. Both varieties are going to be soothing on the stomach, but there are some differences that may make one more suitable than the other.

Loose camomile contains more of the flower, so it is going to be more potent. I'd advise loose camomile when you're going through a particularly bad flare or when you have time to sit and steep it. The downside is that unless you buy a cup with an inbuilt steeper, you're going to need a lot of paraphernalia to extract the tea from the flowers. So, this isn't ideal if you're on the road or wanting to drink a cup at work.

Pressed camomile tea is more practical because the teabags are very slimline. The downside is that because you're not getting all of the flowers seeping into the liquid, the strength is reduced. Though, I do drink several cups of pressed camomile a day, especially after meals or if I'm feeling stressed. I've also found different brands to be hit and miss, with some camomile tea brands being really weak. I also add two teabags if I'm having a flare and don't have access to loose camomile.

Camomile Tea FAQ

I've answered some of your most common questions about how to make camomile tea below. If you need any further help, I'd suggest finding a great independent tea store or contacting the manufacturer of your chosen tea brand directly. Just remember not to boil the life out of it, and you'll generally be fine.

Do I Add Milk To Camomile Tea?

No! Camomile is a flower. You aren't looking to soften the tannins of regular tea and coffee. It's not the same type of drink. At a push, you may add some honey, though I'd personally opt for ultra high grade healing honey so that it offers some benefit beyond a slightly sweeter taste. Watch your sugar intake with honey also.

How Many Cups Of Camomile Tea Should I Drink Per Day?

That is entirely up to you. I would drink it after each meal or whenever I felt highly stressed in my job. Camomile tea doesn't contain caffeine, so it's not going to make you hyper alert or give you a racing heartbeat as too much caffeine would. Start with 1-3 cups per day and see how you feel. You'll know if you fancy more or less.

Who Should Not Drink Camomile Tea?

Anyone who has allergies to camomile or any plants belonging to the daisy family should not consume camomile tea. If you have any other health indications or concerns, you don't need me to tell you to check in with your doctor before trying any new food or health regime. You could also try an allergy test if you suspect you have a camomile allergy, though from what I've found, this is exceptionally rare.

4.7 PROBIOTICS

Similar to how a daily stretching routine, watching your posture and finally giving into yoga or pilates can help keep your spine in check, we also need to take daily steps to keep our gut in order too. One of the simplest ways you can do so is to take a good quality probiotic each day, and no, not just when you are feeling 'off' but commit to doing so each day from this point on.

Ultimately, your whole health hinges on the health of your gut, as it is responsible for absorbing nutrients that feed your body. Yet, the sad part is that nobody will tell you about probiotics, even though they are kind of essential for your gut health in general, let alone if you have GERD.

In fact, even going through countless doctors trying to get an answer to my own GERD symptoms, probiotics were only mentioned very late in the game when I really pushed for something I could do to help myself, having not even been given as much as a diet plan or an explanation of my symptoms.

So what are probiotics, and why are they worth your attention?

Your body, and more specifically your gut, contains a lot of bacteria. Now, naturally, when you hear the word 'bacteria', you picture the bad type, but our gut actually contains good bacteria too, which we need. Only sometimes through reasons such as a poor diet, stress, illness or even due to taking antibiotics, the level of good bacteria in our gut can be out of whack, with bad bacteria overtaking instead.

The simplest way of explaining probiotics is that they boost the good levels of bacteria in your gut to help outweigh the bad. Probiotics contain live organisms that directly add to the population of healthy microbes in your gut, and we don't pay as far as much attention to gut bacteria as we should. So now is the time to start!

Probiotics come in the form of tablet capsules, live yoghurt and milk drinks. However, an important point to note is that with 'live' probiotics, the number of organisms will decrease over time. That's not to say you shouldn't take yoghurt or milk forms of probiotics, but that if you have GERD, you may have to double up or opt for a premium capsule version to ensure you are really getting the number of good bacteria needed to make a difference.

Also, probiotics are not the type of thing you can take once, and bingo, you're cured. But, they are something you should take every day to ensure your gut has everything it needs to thrive. It may take several weeks to start to notice a difference. I know that's disheartening, but when you consider you're trying to undo a chronic problem, even when you're doing all the right things, it can take time and a determined effort to get the balance back in your favour. But, compared with continuing as you are, you'll be so glad you stuck with it.

I personally take Probio7 capsules. As well as being stomach acid resistant (meaning the nutrients will actually reach the gut), they are gluten and dairy free. This makes them suitable for those with related dietary issues as well as vegans. The capsules can be consumed whole, or you can twist them apart and stir the powder into a smoothie.

I was so impressed with these tablets I reached out to the company, and they kindly provided a quote for my book about their product. We also sat down for a chat to talk about all things

GERD, the effect of stress on the gut as well as probiotics. You can catch that on their YouTube channel if you are interested.

Otherwise, here is what Probio7's head of nutrition Rebecca Traylen has to say about the role of probiotics, and in particular Probio7 probiotics in helping GERD (we revert to British English spelling of 'esophagus' here).

Probio7 is a probiotic supplement containing billions of well-researched strains of friendly bacteria as well as natural fibres to help support your gut health.

Your gut health is home to trillions of bacteria and plays a number of important roles in digestion, immunity, skin, mood and sleep. This delicate ecosystem can become unbalanced (otherwise known as dysbiosis) through diet, illness, medication and stress, which can lead to the development of certain digestive symptoms, including acid reflux.

Heartburn is a common symptom of acid reflux whereby acid travels in the wrong direction, up from your stomach and into your oesophagus. Unlike your stomach, your oesophagus isn't designed for this acid and, as a result, triggers a burning sensation in your chest – otherwise known as heartburn. Heartburn can often come about once you eat too much food, as this creates an unequal pressure between your stomach and oesophagus. When this pressure reaches a certain level, it opens your oesophageal sphincter – this acts as a door between your stomach and oesophagus – and allows acid to flow upwards into the oesophagus.

Some people can experience these symptoms more frequently. This is known as gastro-oesophageal reflux disease (GERD or sometimes termed GORD). Some people are more genetically susceptible to GERD, there is also a connection between H.pylori infection and GERD. Some people may also experience heartburn without experiencing acid reflux, this is termed 'functional heartburn' and can be related to a dysfunction between the gut and the brain. Certain diet and lifestyle factors can decrease your risk of GERD, including the use of probiotics.

Probio7 delivers billions of good bacteria to your gut microbiome to help balance this ecosystem, remove pathogenic microorganisms by strengthening the gut barrier and reduce inflammation in the gut.

I want to thank Rebecca and the Probio7 team for their help in making sure we fully explain the role of probiotics in our gut health.

I've had folks from Canada and other countries write to me that they can't get hold of this specific brand. Probio7 is available outside of the UK, so it's certainly worth trying to find it. I personally buy the advanced formula, which is slightly more expensive but to be honest, it's money well spent when your gut remains healthy, and you don't experience any flare-ups.

If you can't find Probio7 - don't panic! Instead, head to your nearest health food store or pharmacist, and ask them for their best probiotic that you can afford.

Here's a checklist I put together for you to consider:

Probiotic Checklist

- How much bacteria does it contain?
- What strains of bacteria does it contain?
- Is the formula stomach acid resistant so that it will actually reach the gut properly?
- Does it need to be refrigerated?
- Does it contain anything I'm allergic to? (if applicable, for example, gluten)
- Do I need to consult my doctor first? (pregnancy, severe allergies etc.)

- What are the usage directions?
- Is this brand reputable, and are there good reviews?
- How am I going to remember to take it every day?

For the uninitiated, the cost of probiotics can seem steep at £20-£40 ($27-$55) for a really decent brand for around a month's supply. However, I personally think it's 100% worth the investment. Plus, if you've stopped buying fast food and cleaned up your diet (if that was ever you), it actually shouldn't leave you out of pocket when you think about it. I also don't think you can really put a price on good gut health, especially if you've been suffering for so long.

Also, if you are on or have recently taken antibiotics, the good bacteria in your gut is going to be wiped out anyway, which is why the instructions will often state to double up your dosage for a couple of weeks until optimum levels of good bacteria return.

Take the probiotics as instructed on the box or bottle, as each brand or type differs slightly. For example, Probio7 recommends taking a capsule with breakfast, or if you are on antibiotics, to take a capsule with a meal around 2-4 hours after taking your antibiotic. In general, most probiotic manufacturers will advise double dosage if you're on antibiotics, so always study the labels carefully.

You can also use live yoghurt or probiotic milk drink to soothe a flare or before exercising to give you energy for your workout without gravity inducing a flare. So yes, you can mix and match your probiotics as you see fit.

Some people may experience digestive discomfort as they get used to probiotics. In which case, provided you don't have any allergies to any of the ingredients, it's worth sticking with probiotics to see if the symptoms ease. After all, if you're dealing with mostly bad bacteria, you need to let the good bacteria come in and do its thing, and this takes time to do.

Another positive point about probiotics is that they can be instrumental in helping other conditions, including skin complaints such as acne or rosacea. Now, that's not to say taking probiotics will *definitely cure any certain condition*, but, given what we know about the importance of gut health on our whole body and even our mental health, it stands to reason that by improving our gut health, the effects could be wide reaching in the most positive of ways. I personally notice they make my skin glow and keep my GERD at bay over the long term, which I'm pretty delighted about.

Probiotics For Travel

Have you ever noticed that despite the point of booking a trip somewhere is to destress, travelling actually is one of the most stressful things ever?

Booking travel tickets, sorting an itinerary, trying to get all of your work done before you leave, scheduling an appointment with your wax therapist where you will actually pay to be tortured (ok that last one is just me!). In all seriousness, I don't think anyone ever talks about the amount of metal capacity it takes to organise everything for a trip, which can actually get things off on the wrong foot.

Travel can stress your gut mentally and physically, so it's essential to prepare for travel by continuing to take probiotics before, during and after your trip. Some companies (including Probio7) also make probiotics that have been specifically formulated for travel. But, any probiotic is going to be better than none.

Prebiotics Vs Probiotics

Both prebiotics and probiotics sound very similar, and given the lack of education around gut health, it's very easy to get confused between the two. It's not a competition, as both prebiotics and probiotics are beneficial for gut health, and you may want to start investing in each to maximise your results. In fact, some experts have said that prebiotics are the food for probiotics, which is a great way to think about it.

Prebiotics are types of dietary fibre that help feed the friendly bacteria in our gut and are most commonly found in any foods that contain complex carbohydrates such as fibre or resistant starch. Interestingly, these substances are not directly digestible by the body, though they pass through the digestive system to become food for the digestive system itself.

Probiotics are live strains of bacteria that help our digestive system and directly add to the friendly microbes in our gut. We need good bacteria for our gut, yet it's easy for our good bacteria to become depleted. Hence, probiotics work to increase the levels of good bacteria to hopefully outweigh the bad bacteria.

Some supplements also contain both prebiotics and probiotics, and these are known as symbiotics. The goal of symbiotics is to increase the levels of good bacteria in your gut while simultaneously providing a source of energy for the good bacteria.

New to all things prebiotics and probiotics? Both are going to help to keep your gut in check, so if you have GERD you need to be reading up on them. As well as consulting your doctor, any gut or dietary expert should be able to help you. Also, a pharmacist or trusted health food store may be able to offer free advice. Just don't let it be one of those things you forget about, when your gut needs all the help it can get right now.

4.8 REINTRODUCING FOODS

As we know, the focus with a GERD friendly diet is alkaline foods, excluding both unhealthy processed food as well as anything acidic, even if it may be a healthy acid such as tomatoes, citrus fruits or spicy food.

However, eating alkaline is quite restrictive, which is why although eating alkaline from this point on as much as possible is always a good idea, at some stage, you will need to look at reintroducing acids back into your diet too.

This is so you are receiving an adequate amount of nutrition. Also, it's important that you learn to enjoy food again, especially as food is a cornerstone of so much of our lives, including social occasions. So it's definitely a case of making smarter choices, so you never find yourself back here, rather than never touching acidic food ever again. Life is too short for that!

The problem is that restrictive eating to cure your GERD can in turn cause an issue. It's tricky because you can't get out of cutting out foods which are going to trigger you, so you have to do it; otherwise, your condition won't improve - especially if your diet has always been acid heavy. But at the same time, you need to also be conscious of slowly reintroducing foods when the time is right.

So don't think the work is over when you're feeling better by any means, because you need to complete that last step to get you back to eating a balanced and varied diet.

You may want to consult a therapist or nutritionist if you have difficulty in this area with your mental health. The last thing I'd want for anyone is to heal from GERD, only to develop an eating disorder or any other dietary related problem. I know it's a lot to think about, but at least by being thorough, you're going to have a better chance of regaining normality.

I definitely went through a phase where I was scared to eat certain foods because of the memory of how it triggered my symptoms. That's why I made a conscious effort to revisit these foods as soon as I was well enough.

If you think about it, it's totally normal to have such a reaction. You've gone through something massive with your stomach, and it's going to take time to mentally and physically resume regular activity. But, you also have to know when you're feeling fit and strong, meaning it's safe to broaden your diet again.

As for when the time is right, that is down to you and your gut. It's definitely going to take a few weeks of alkaline foods and high strength probiotics for your stomach to be in a much better position. For me, it took a few months because my GERD was extremely uncontrolled, and I hadn't had any help with my diet plan. But if I had known to avoid acidic foods and reduce stress, I'm sure this timeframe would have been a lot less.

So my advice is to give it a few weeks and then check in with yourself. When you wake up, do you feel a sense of relief that you are starting to feel better, or does your stomach still burn like hell? This will tell you whether you can start taking those first steps with *mildly* acidic foods or whether you need to continue as you are for just a little longer.

In the background, I am assuming you are working on reducing your stress levels, exercising and sleeping well. If any of these things are out of whack, it's going to delay your recovery, so make sure you're covering all bases here.

For hiatal hernia patients, yout recovery really needs to be planned between you and your doctor since diet and probiotics alone aren't enough to fix physical obstructions. So, if you do end up having surgery, your medical team needs to guide you on how to resume eating again, including what to eat and getting the balance right.

But assuming your GERD has been caused by diet, stress or an unhealthy lifestyle in general, test the water with a small amount of food that previously would have been too acidic, such as a tomato pasta dish. **Do not head straight for a greasy burger or a fatty dessert.** If, with every bite, you're feeling hungry and it's not causing any immediate burning, then this is a good sign.

Have a cup of camomile tea afterwards, and see how everything feels. If you didn't receive an almighty flare, then you know at least whatever you tried can now be included in your new menu. It's a gradual process to return to a healthy and balanced diet, so go easy on yourself and don't expect miracles.

If whatever you tried to eat did cause a flare, consider what that food was and whether it was a healthy option or not. If you went straight for that greasy burger or spicy curry, you didn't read what I just advised above, which is unfortunate. Otherwise, if you are being good, then you may simply need a bit more time on the alkaline diet with daily probiotics.

Obviously, take the time to eat your meal correctly regardless and do not overeat so that you don't inadvertently cause a flare-up. Remember, our stomach has a limited size, and if we overeat, it's going to stretch, be uncomfortable and trigger an attack. You must never let yourself get to that point.

4.9 BRINGING A GERD FLARE UNDER CONTROL

Skip to this section of the book anytime you're in a jam with your GERD and need to know what to do about it.

I have covered the issue of bringing a GERD flare-up under control in various ways throughout. But I also thought it would be handy to address it directly in its own section in case you are struggling right this second and need a quick fix.

So long as your GERD is not due to an anatomical defect, you should find some relief from the toolkit below. If your GERD is stress or anxiety related, I would recommend steps such as a walk in the fresh air, a hot bath, exercise, listening to a calming playlist etc.

Obviously, chronic anxiety or stress will require a more targeted approach which you're going to need to get on top of, possibly with specialist help or the support of friends and family.

Without further ado, to quickly bring a GERD flare-up under control, I'd encourage you to try one or a combination of the following:

- Alkaline green juice/smoothie
- Kefir (plain)

- Camomile tea
- Probiotic milk
- Probiotic tablets
- Probiotic yoghurt

Alkaline Green Juice/Smoothie

Best for: When you have woken up with symptoms, before a workout or if you are struggling with your appetite.

If you are looking to settle your stomach from a purely pH basis, one of the quickest ways to do so is to get some alkaline fluids in there.

Some suitable ingredients to make either a juice or a smoothie (be sure to choose the right combination that work best in a juicer or a blender) include a base of either oat or almond milk with the likes of celery, spinach, avocado, cucumber, spirulina, acai and bananas.

Double check the pH of any ingredient before adding it in if you're not sure. You can also empty in a probiotic capsule for added clout (Probio7 capsules can be broken in half for this very reason).

P.S: Don't consume this one if you're having a flare-up because you've overeaten, especially the likes of avocado which is extremely filling. Wait until you naturally feel hungry again, because you must let your stomach empty of its own accord.

Camomile Tea

Best for: After eating or anytime you are feeling stressed or anxious.

Camomile tea ranges from being neutral to alkaline, depending on the variety you opt for. It was instrumental in my GERD recovery, particularly the loose leaf variety, which is the most potent type. It's also great if you're feeling highly stressed or anxious, helping to relieve your GERD from another angle than just the contents of your stomach.

Kefir (Plain)

Best for: As an alternative to breakfast, or if you've eaten a small meal that's given you a flare therefore consuming this yoghurt type drink won't cause you to feel overfull, but it will help to settle your symptoms.

Kefir is a fermented milk drink that helps to fan the flames of a flare-up. I recently ate some food that I didn't realise was going to be as greasy as it was, causing heartburn symptoms to pop up. Within an hour of drinking a plain kefir drink I felt much better and within a couple of hours my appetite returned to normal.

Probiotics

Best for: Adding a soothing liquid to your gut that will also help boost your digestion in general.

In the immediate point of a flare, probiotic milks are excellent, followed by probiotic yoghurts. The tablet versions are based for long term GERD relief and should be consumed daily.

Finally, if you're having a GERD flare right now check your breathing and your pulse. If your pulse is elevated and you aren't taking deep breaths, you need to address this immediately, because this isn't going to help your flare regardless of what you eat. In fact, being in such a heightened state could have even triggered your flare in the first place.

Go outside if you can and get some fresh air. Inhale some essential oils and listen to some calming music. Talk out any issues with a friend, and get your stress under control. Or even hit the gym if you're really worked up. You've got this.

5.0 STRESS

Humans were designed to be able to handle stress to a certain degree. As hunter-gatherers, we would occasionally encounter physical situations that would make us either fight or flight. The problem is that this extreme level of adrenaline which allowed us to be able to act quickly to diffuse whatever situation was in front of us, was only ever designed to be temporary. In today's world, more of us are chronically stressed than ever, meaning we are technically permanently stuck in this state of fight or flight. We're on edge, tense, nervous, agitated, stressed or anxious too often. It's a complete overload.

We've established that the mind and the gut are closely connected, an example being when you're nervous, and you get butterflies in your stomach. Or when you've had bad news, and you lose your appetite. Stress along with anxiety and depression can manifest itself in many ways, and for some, this results in a GERD flare-up. For many people, stress is the root cause of their GERD altogether.

When you're not feeling well, this can also be stressful in itself, especially in the age of being able to Google your symptoms.

It's difficult to tell you not to stress when you are utterly exasperated with GERD. But, I will say that unless you get your stress under control, you are going to have a problem recovering.

When we are stressed, our bodies are stuck in that 'high alert' mode. We don't take the time to eat properly. We're more likely to eat bad food, smoke, drink and whatever else we do that's bad for our health to relieve the pressure.

Unfortunately, our bodies are living creatures, and they don't respond well when they aren't getting what they need. It's crazy how that simple fact is news to so many people.

No two people are the same in terms of how they handle stress. Some people are completely unfazed in the most heightened of situations. Others are incredibly anxious all of the time to the point they struggle to leave their homes. Neither of these are actually healthy scenarios. So, the approach you take here needs to be tailored to you, the individual.

I do think talking helps, but it really depends on who you have to talk to. Some people are absolutely useless at listening, which only makes things worse. Many people might not care. So, it's always good to surround yourself with the right people and don't be afraid to remove toxic influences from your life (yes, even if you are related). If your stress is particularly bad, it's worth looking into therapy. Now, I know some people will automatically shriek when I say that, especially if you're British.

Often the image is that to talk about how you are feeling it means you are weak. Only, this view is not only outdated but incredibly harmful too. If your mental health isn't looking very rosy and you don't have anyone you feel comfortable talking to about it, then you must, for your own sake, find someone to talk to. It doesn't matter what age or gender you are either - do not bottle this up as GERD will be the least of your problems if you do.

As I mentioned, we spend 90% of our time indoors. We are not spending enough time away from screens, immersed in nature. In fact, when was the last time you took a walk in a nice park or by the sea? The problem is if we treat our bodies with the same regard as our technology and not the living, breathing beings we actually are, then we begin to suffer. Every single person needs time to relax and destress. It's not an 'airy fairy' concept, nor is it selfish - it's a necessity.

Personally, one of my favourite activities is to go for a deep tissue massage, such as a Swedish massage. To set the scene, you are in a room with calming music, which already starts to slow your breathing pattern. All of your knots are worked out of your back, particularly where we carry a lot of tension around the neck and shoulders. Our muscles also produce waste products, and massages help to flush out these toxins from the muscles to oxygenate them and improve movement. You are required to do nothing but lay on a table for 60 minutes, and similar to being on a plane, you'd be surprised how de-stressing it is when nobody can contact you or ask you to do anything for those precious few minutes. In today's hectic world - we need this time to be able to recharge our batteries.

It only takes a few minutes of a (good!) massage until you completely forget all of your worries. It makes your mind switch off. When you've been concentrating on your ailments, I can't tell you how beneficial this is. Some spas even have infrared saunas you can go in beforehand, which makes the massage even more effective and really promotes healing within the body. This is exactly the type of activity I'd recommend with GERD, especially on the weekend after a stressful week at work.

So that you feel comfortable with your GERD, I suggest avoiding large meals, especially 3-4 hours before you go in. Drink plenty of water afterwards (they usually bring you a glass) to flush those toxins out.

I once had a massage at Massage Revolution in Santa Monica. I'd just left my job, and my GERD was still giving me trouble because I hadn't healed yet plus my neck was busted. Their massages are targeted to chronic pain, and they are incredibly skilled in muscles and trigger points. Anyway, when I came out, it was hilarious because I actually sounded like I had the flu because of all the toxins the massage released out of my muscles! It's proof that massages really do work.

Of course not everyone is going to want to try a spa, and that's okay. But you do need to find another healthy way to let go of stress and negative energy, such as exercise. I have written a section on exercising with GERD, which goes into greater detail. However, exercise is something you should try and do at least two to three times a week.

If you have a lot of stress from your job, then waking up early to do some stretches or even go for a walk if you live near a nice spot can help. Though for me, nothing beats stress exercise wise compared to getting on a treadmill. I really do think 'sweating it out' can really work wonders, and an added benefit is sometimes the extra energy you exert can help with your appetite too. Remember, if you are struggling to eat, don't force it, just be sure to stay hydrated, especially after exercise.

Another way to deal with your stress is quite simply to get to the root cause of it. This is going to mean different things to different people. On a basic level, sometimes we just put too much pressure on ourselves. We don't hit the brakes when we should. Or, we make our lives way too complicated. Or we just spread ourselves too thinly.

As someone in her thirties, let me tell you, the societal pressure to have everything 'figured out' by now is immense. You're supposed to hit all these milestones, and if you don't, then there's something 'wrong' with you. Actually taking the time to step back and realise it's okay to carve your own path and go at your own pace is life-changing. I know that whatever life stage you are at, you'll probably have your own expectations from society and yourself that you're trying to live up to. In reality, what you need to do is just breathe. Yes, be motivated and determined in life but not to the point where it's giving you serious health conditions, you know? It's just not going to get you anywhere.

If it helps, then write down your top stressors. Try and figure out a way to deal with each thing that is stressing you out in a way that's proactive but most of all plausible.

Let's take money as an example, which is a source of stress for most people unless you're Jeff Bezos, I guess. We spend most of our time at work trying to earn money. You can't do much without it, and to be honest, it practically rules us. The stress it can create when we don't have enough or if you are in debt can cripple our emotional wellbeing. So, if that sounds like you, it's definitely worth getting some advice and working out how to move forward.

While sorting your stress won't cure your GERD on its own (though to be honest, it might for some of you), reducing yours will significantly contribute to your body's ability to heal. That's because instead of your body thinking to itself, 'right, I better stay on high alert here', - it can divert the enormous amount of energy and resources your stress is taking up to sorting other stuff out, including your GERD.

After I walked out of my job, I went to see a therapist because I did not like what the job had done to my mental state, particularly how negative I became. Also, it's really not a good look to quit your job by telling your boss what you thought of the company in a brutal five page letter. Even if it needed to be said, I never wanted to be in the position again where I flipped out like that.

I told my therapist how I wanted to manage my stress better. Then, she did something which I felt uncomfortable with, which was to share other client stories with me in acute detail. It's supposed to be confidential! At that point, I wanted to run for the hills, and after session two, I did. But before that point, she told me how her clients included local nurses who had mixed medications up, and company directors who had walked out of their jobs. Her response was: "If only they had come to see me first, I could have given them the coping skills they need!"

My perspective on this is, why do we need to learn such extreme coping, no scratch, that more like survival skills just to earn a paycheck? If a nurse is giving out the wrong medication and harming patients, then either she hasn't had adequate training or is quite frankly overworked. Why must the blame always get shifted solely on the person who acts out? It's like yeah 'Susan' you let the side down, you've brought this hospital into disrepute, it's your fault the patient is taking legal action because you gave out the wrong pills. What about all the crap the employer and the system put on her in the first place that meant she was unable to function properly and therefore made a mistake? But no, people just want to stand there with their pitchforks instead. Nobody is stopping to think. In some cases, I think most people lack that capacity. They just want blood regardless.

Why when someone takes issue with any system, are you immediately labelled as a weak, millennial snowflake? It's gaslighting at its finest, I tell you.

So I will say to all those who are in stressful jobs, whether it be from the work itself, the culture or the management, honestly just get the hell out. No, not because you're a quitter (please don't quit in the way I did either), but because your life is going to end at some point, and if it's making you ill, it's not acceptable. Even though society tells you it is, it's not. There are other jobs out there you can do where you will be appreciated, but most importantly, your mental health will be intact.

Make sure you do speak to someone in between jobs, so you don't take the baggage with you either. Looking back, I definitely think I did that, especially as every time the phone rang in my new job, I would freeze. I mean, the 'worst' the call could have been about is someone wanting to enquire about some marketing. But in my head, it was a grieving parent on the other end of the phone. Or someone who was going to threaten us for printing a story.

I did end up trying therapy again, although not for too long because the sessions were £120 ($150) per week which I couldn't justify budget wise. However, while I was there, my therapist did make quite a few observations that I found really helped me.

Just for context, this therapist worked a lot in the London corporate scene, and was also involved in the mental rehabilitation of the Grenfell Tower victims. So, she understands trauma just as she does general working environments.

When I was talking about struggling with the nature of the case details we were privy to, particularly involving the deaths of children or horrendous accidents etc., she bluntly asked me why no training was given before being exposed to such details, nor any debriefs arranged for the more traumatic cases. Instead, we had to get on with the next story and the next, churning everything out to hit all our requirements, while being overworked, understaffed and underpaid. Remember, I wasn't even a qualified journalist!

Well when you look at it from that perspective, *of course* burnout was inevitable. I'd only blamed myself up to that point for not being resilient enough in the job. Yet here was an independent expert actually telling me it was basically unavoidable that I walked out like that.

Gaining some fresh perspective on your stress or even previous sources of stress can really unlock so much. Even if you just have a catch up with friends or family members. Compared with keeping everything in your own head, it's really beneficial to hear other takes on what you went through sometimes.

It's not an easy discussion, and you may think about how you should have done better, but you'll also learn a lot more about yourself from doing so. Sometimes we blame ourselves for everything when we really shouldn't.

5.1 RECOGNISING YOU'RE STRESSED

It's my belief that most people are in denial about their stress or that 'coping' with high levels of stress is seen as some sort of term of endearment. The reality is, as I stated before, that yes, humans are designed to handle acute stress to some degree, but not to a chronic level.

It's not how we were designed, and yet it's something we have a huge problem admitting to, let alone properly tackling. This could not be more true within a work environment, where so often it's a source of shame to admit you are stressed, despite the fact it is often the environment itself and the impossible setup of the company and unrealistic expectations that cause the stress in the first place.

So, there's definitely stress to consider from multiple angles, both on a personal level in terms of yourself, your home life, friends and family etc., and if you work, within your professional life too.

Symptoms of stress include:

- Avoiding others
- Becoming easily agitated
- Changes in appetite
- Chest pain
- Dry mouth

- Feeling overwhelmed
- Frequent colds
- Headaches
- Inability to focus
- Insomnia
- Loss of libido
- Low energy
- Low self-esteem
- Nervous behaviours (nail biting, fidgeting, pacing)
- Procrastination (avoiding responsibilities)
- Racing thoughts
- Struggling to relax
- Teeth grinding
- Upset stomach
- Use of alcohol, cigarettes or drugs

Does any of the above sound familiar? You might just be stressed!

It's going to require a huge effort to get on top of your stress, but now is probably the best time to do so since you're also experiencing GERD.

Bearing in mind tomorrow is a clean slate, as we mentioned, what changes can you make in the morning to fix your stress for good? From simple changes such as a nice walk to more drastic changes to your health or lifestyle - reducing your stress is now in your hands.

5.2 TOXIC ENVIRONMENTS

Something that dawned on me recently is that we don't really talk about toxic work environments and the impact this can have on employees. In part, this is due to the fear of looking unprofessional or it affecting future work opportunities.

Now, just because your boss can grate on you or be annoying, that doesn't mean they are a bad boss, so it's important not to tar all bosses with the same brush. However, the ugly truth is there are a lot of people working in managerial roles that do not possess actual people skills. The problem is, so many of these poor personal traits soon infiltrate the rest of the team and ultimately the whole company.

Some general examples may include:

- Unclear communication
- Unrealistic expectations
- Constantly changing goalposts
- Bullying or humiliation tactics
- Narcissistic or top-down leadership
- A reluctance to approve time off
- Deliberately not having enough staff to complete the workload leading to employee burnout
- Deadlines always taking priority over emotional wellbeing
- No focus on developing company culture

Whether you recognise these signs in your workplace, or if you are dealing with a toxic situation in your personal life - protecting your energy is everything. If you're in an environment that's confrontational, mean spirited or a general energy vacuum, it can trigger a flare-up of your GERD.

Now you might wonder why, in a book about GERD, would someone be harping on about mental wellbeing. Well, remember, the simple answer is the brain and gut are intrinsically linked. So, while your GERD may well be caused by a hernia, pregnancy or another unrelated cause, it's impossible to heal fully without considering all possible triggers including your mental wellbeing.

If our bodies are stuck in a state of high emotion, all its resources are diverted into fight or flight. Is healing your GERD going to be top of the agenda? It's probably not even *on* the agenda if the situation is that bad. So, there's no point gulping down celery juice if you then have a huge argument with your partner or dread washes over you going into work. It's time to make the connection because healing from any condition is always going to require a 360 approach.

So, it may well be the case your triggers include your partner, family, friends, coworkers or neighbours.

In many cases, people don't even realise they are being subjected to toxic abuse, especially in the case of narcissism as just one example. I know that word is bandied around a lot, and just because someone you know drains you, that doesn't mean they are a narcissist. But it's worth educating yourself on all forms of toxic behaviour so you know the signs.

Sometimes, you have to cut all ties to protect your energy, yes, even if you are related to that person or even married to them, or if this job you're in is supposed to be a golden opportunity.

If the issue cannot be reasoned with, then unless you remove yourself from the situation, it will never improve. So have a think whether any of this applies to you.

5.3 WORK STRESS

The UK mental health charity Mind estimates that work is the most stressful factor in people's lives, with 10% of 18-24 year olds reporting suicidal thoughts directly attributed to work stress.

Undoubtedly, any kind of toxic environment within your place of work specifically is going to lead to stress. Work stress is a complex one, because all jobs have some element of stress to them. But where do you draw the line between acceptable and unacceptable?

Also, a job isn't something we do just for fun. It's our way of earning a living, and for most people providing for their family. With so much attached to your job, even if the demands have crossed well into the 'unacceptable' territory, you're probably reluctant to leave it.

We're also conditioned into thinking that part of 'making it' in life is pushing ourselves beyond our limits. Can we just backtrack for a second, and actually consider that analogy in greater depth?

I mentioned how my job pretty much triggered my GERD in the first place. Given we all need to work to survive, there's a high chance your GERD is being triggered by your work, or rather your work conditions.

Here's the thing, when you go to work for an employer you are there to serve them. It's not about you, it's about them getting what they need done. I get this entirely, I'm not lazy, workshy or any other adjective that gets thrown at my age group whenever we raise a genuinely valid point these days.

The problem is far too many employers push this as far as possible until you either bend into their shape and compromise who you are or simply break.

I do think it's a problem when you dedicate your best ideas and well, your whole life to a company that doesn't care about you. For example, I've seen sickening examples where loyal employees have been denied time off for their kid's cancer treatment or their parents funeral. How did society come to this?

I also know of far too many people whose whole identity consists of their job, when actually the two things should never be that closely entwined. Why? Firstly there is more to life, yes even if you love your job. Most importantly, if your job is your whole world, you're far more likely to make allowances if the treatment of you and your colleagues slides. In too many cases, employers know this.

When people call out unacceptable behaviour, there is sadly always a backlash. But if people don't make a stand, how will society ever improve? Why can't employees come to work and fulfil their duties without being subjected to bullying and harassment? Why is unpaid overtime being written into people's contracts when you didn't sign up to volunteer but to earn a living and pay your bills?

The simple truth is because most companies do not value their employees. When your employees are human beings but you treat them like robots, there's a disconnect. On a lighter level, it's someone thinking the job isn't for them, and that they eventually want to move into a different career. But when it's deeply systemic, it can have catastrophic implications for that person's health and wellbeing.

The most ironic thing is that if an employee feels happy and well supported in their role, it will show in their work. The applicable (I'm well aware it's not everyone) employers think that by treating their staff like something they stepped on, it will bring them into line. All it does is cause tension and bitter resentment, not to mention a high turnover of staff. Surely that's actually costing your company more money in the long term?

Once at another job interview, I was asked why I left my GERD inducing job given it was such a good opportunity. I replied that I found the job stressful, especially given the abuse you'd get from the public. The fact that constant redundancies meant they weren't just trimming the fat, but were cutting deeply into the bone. Or words to that effect.

Now, you might be thinking, 'oh god why would you be so honest'. The thing is, I really hate how at job interviews you have to lie. For example, when they ask why you want to work there. The real answer is to pay your bills. But instead, you have to go into a long, flowery appraisal of their company you pieced together the night before off Wikipedia. I know it's what you're supposed to do, but then the very first interaction I'm having is a complete lie, so how is that 'right and proper' over telling the truth? Why do job interviews so often feel like a giant ego stroking exercise? I just want to get to work.

As you can predict, I didn't get the job. This is a snippet of the email I got as part of my rejection letter: "*A point of constructive criticism for you…Although I encourage honesty being the best policy in an interview setting, I would suggest that 'being too stressful' is not the best reason to provide for the leaving of a previous role. I think it'd be fair to say that every employer in the country deem their company to be somewhere they need their staff to be able to cope with a certain amount of pressure and this statement does not convey that notion.*"

Just to be a bitch, I didn't edit out their use of ellipses intended to create suspense, which Jay Rayner said is one of the worst grammatical mistakes you can make as a writer. Hence it's the only '...' you'll find in this entire book. I digress.

Anyway, on the same day I received that email, there was a story in the very publication I worked for because someone had threatened to shoot a former colleague of mine and the case had gone to court. Only, I'm female and I'm a millennial. So, even if I had replied back with a link to the article demonstrating not a single fragment of what I said was exaggerated, it still wouldn't have been enough. I'm still in the wrong for saying excessive stress to the point where your mental health is being seriously compromised isn't how a business should be run. I stand by that point vehemently, even if nobody would employ me for saying it. To be honest, if they truly feel that way then I'm glad they wouldn't. Because you're simply shifting the blame onto the person calling out the stress, rather than those creating it. I'm sorry, but that's just not right.

When you hold a mirror up to bad employers or toxic workplace culture in general, those who perpetuate the behaviour you call out cannot deal with the beast they have created or at least contributed to. It's rife, and so no wonder a lot of people develop GERD from workplace stress. Please join up the dots here!

I'll give you another example. A few years back I worked in retail. My job was to go around different department stores and supermarkets promoting fragrance launches. Sometimes I'd cover beauty counters too where I'd advise customers, colour match them to products etc.

I had a couple of occasions where the manager would come darting over telling me I had to unload stock in the warehouse or even take over work from their colleagues. I would tell them that that wasn't in my contract, nor was I trained or insured to do any of what they just asked me to do. All of a sudden, it's "you're not a team player", or "you're not proactive", or better still, "why did you even turn up today then?" This was after I got up at 5am, put on a full face of makeup and travelled two hours on a bus where it was so cold you'd see your breath when you exhaled to do that shift. Yet no, now 'I'm not committed'. Erm.

Basically, if I don't put myself in danger by using machinery I have no training in, and I don't do the work that is actually the responsibility of others, I'm not a valued employee. Even though it would be illegal for me to do what they are asking of me, and a huge risk for their company if I had an accident because I was made to do something potentially very dangerous I wasn't insured or trained to do. I've seen companies forced out of business for similar industrial accidents, and it also ruins the life of the person involved if they can't work again. One of my current clients owns an insurance comparison website - I get paid to know this stuff now, believe me it happens.

While working for the same company for a store across the street, I was pulled aside again to do stuff that wasn't in my contract. Every day, the staff had to get a certain number of credit card signups otherwise they'd be taken into the office and yelled at by the manager. They'd come back shaking looking really upset. They were falling behind in their signups. So they asked me if I would stop what I was doing, go up to customers and persuade them to get a credit card to get the manager off their backs.

At the time, I was working for a French perfume brand for a new product launch. I had to have training to be able to do this job, so that I could explain all the fragrance notes to the customers. My role was to hand samples out and get customers to purchase the product, as well as assist with other fragrance brands when they were busy. I worked for the agency itself and not the store I was placed in.

Yet, I was suddenly being asked to stop my role, and do something I morally disagree with, which is to get people into debt, as the interest rates on these cards were abhorrent. I previously ran a money saving website FYI, hence I would never in a million years encourage such a scheme. So I refused.

They would take great delight in a customer not having good English, because they wouldn't fully understand what they were signing up for. The customers just thought they were getting a discount on their shopping. There's no way I was going to be a part of that.

The department store has since gone out of business, perhaps because relying on commission for credit card sign ups is not a sustainable business model? I bet there's thousands of poor sods still trying to pay off the debt they got into from signing up, lured in by the promise of getting 10% off the cost of their eau de piss smelling perfume (depending on which corner of the store you bought from).

Repeat the same scenario for any job, and it's no wonder people are feeling stressed. All the while, they pay you as low as they can get away with.

Now, I'm sure there are far more stressful occupations out there, of course there are but that's not the point of why I just shared all that. Instead, listen to the actual context of what I'm saying here. That is, that it's so, so common to be put into situations you shouldn't be within a work environment. It's seen as a term of endearment to do whatever is asked of you, regardless of whether it's illegal, degrading, immoral or even stuff you're simply not being paid to do in the first place. It doesn't just happen in movies, it's rife in so many different industries.

I cannot tell you how many times the things I have been asked to do vary wildly from my actual contract. Things that were ***never*** mentioned in the interview. I wonder, if I were to stray so far from my job role whether the employer would be so accepting?

The exact nature is going to vary wildly from person to person, but the sentiment remains the same. There's a difference between being a dedicated employee, and going past the point of what's acceptable.

As someone who is self-employed now, me and my clients always have a clear outline of what the project entails. If anything falls outside of the remit, the budget will either have to be renegotiated, or I will politely let them know that's not part of my job description.

But, when you're an employee you can easily get pushed into situations that are wrong without you even realising it. Or sometimes you do realise, but you're too afraid to speak up. So much is riding on you to bring home that paycheck, so you mistakenly think you don't have a choice. If there's a door, then there's always a choice.

If you can relate to any of this, then you aren't going to be able to get a proper handle on your stress until you get out of the situation. Your GERD recovery may well be dependent on reducing your stress from your job, ao it's not something you can ignore.

I know not everyone can just walk out of their jobs. But, I implore you to consider your wellbeing. Believe it or not, there are many other jobs out there you can do that won't give you the 'Sunday night dread'. The problem is, such work environments grind you down to the point where you think you aren't worthy, that no other employer would want you. This just isn't true! So please look at your options, I promise you better exists out there.

Remember, work is likely where you spend the majority of your time. In fact, most people spend more time at work than they do with their families. We know we have to work to be able to pay our bills and take care of all of our responsibilities. So, whatever you do, make sure you're in a job that you're genuinely happy in. If you go to work feeling tense, anxious, stressed etc - your body is trying to tell you something. It might be GERD right now, but what if you stay in this environment? Where will you be in another five years of this crap? Think about it while you still have the chance to change the narrative.

Another way of dealing with work stress, especially if it's general stress that we all face, is to work on your life outside of your job. Consider if you are spending enough of your free time genuinely nourishing your soul.

For example, when was the last time you went for a walk in a park, or visited a new place? Make your free time count. Spend less time scrolling, more time actually living.

How The Office Is Damaging Our Health

We spend 90% of our time indoors. Most of our week is spent working, and for the vast majority of us this is done inside an office. If you've ever observed commuters heading to work in an office on a Monday morning, they don't exactly look thrilled. Why is that?

In Evening Standard article titled '24 ways your office job is destroying your health' they state the following:

- Sitting all day could shave years off your life
- Slouching in an office chair can lead to arthritis and bursitis
- Skipping breakfast messes up your metabolism
- Regularly eating fast food for lunch increases the risk of heart disease
- Long commutes lead to insomnia, high cholesterol and depression

- Recycled air is bad for our lungs
- Working for more than 10 hours a day may lead to a heart attack
- Germs are everywhere in the office
- Uncomfortable work shoes can lead to spinal injuries

The COVID-19 pandemic has also shown a very interesting trend in terms of how we view our office spaces. Here in the UK, many offices remained empty because of social distancing. However, the work still got done by employees at home. Furthermore, many offices (even bigshot central London law firms) actually said remote working was going to be their new normal even after the pandemic. At best, many companies are now adopting a hybrid model whereby employees are only required to come into the office once or twice a week.

As a remote worker myself, I cannot tell you how beneficial a complete 100% avoidance of a physical office space does for your health. GERD wise, not only am I less stressed but I can eat, drink, stretch, go out for a walk etc anytime I like. As long as the work is done to a high standard and on time, the client doesn't care (in a good way). You lose that micromanigerial element of your day which is someone grossly overpaid standing over your shoulder instead of working themselves. It's life-changing I tell you.

Working remotely means more flexibility for parents too, and zero commute. I appreciate it's not for everyone, but I do think remote working should remain an option for those who can make it work. You can't abuse the system, you do have to show a high level of diligence and actually be working.

So, ultimately what the pandemic has shown from a work/life balance perspective is that many people felt unhappy in their old ways. I don't think I've ever worked in a single office job where someone hasn't asked me "If you win the lottery what would you do?".

If you truly love your job, you don't have those thoughts. Even if you do, you don't feel bitter resentment when you see your numbers haven't come up, because you know your life is already great when you enjoy your work.

Stress, unhappiness and self-loathing are toxic forces running through our bodies, and our digestive system is just one of the many casualties of such emotions. If your office job is the source of the problem, then change may be necessary.

5.4 DIGITAL STRESS

Do you remember the days when you could only make a call with a landline phone? We still have ours because certain older relatives 'only use a mobile phone in an emergency'. Give me strength. Anyway, there was a certain beauty of not being constantly connected to the outside world that has now sadly become obsolete.

These days, we are constantly wired to a flurry of notifications whether it's texts, calls, emails, social media or news websites. The problem is that it can be difficult to switch off, not least because the light emitted from our phones stimulates our brain activity. We always feel like we have to be up to date with every single thing happening and it gets overwhelming.

I would like you to think about how much time you spend glued to your phone. Especially if you're the type who takes yours to read on the toilet (sorry, it's a no from me) or if you wake up in the middle and night and check your phone (ok yes, guilty as charged).

The reason is we all need time to switch off, which is impossible to do fully if we are connected to so much incoming information. People think I'm crazy when I tell them this, but I will often go out on walks without my phone. The reason is, I just want to be left alone. I don't want to hear an alert I need to check, nor do I want to be tempted to take a picture of my surroundings even. I just want to get away from my digital device for at least 30 minutes.

There's even digital detox wellness retreats these days, where you head to the forest, camp under the stars and actually have actual conversations with people. I think a fair bit of green juice is involved too. I know that isn't going to be for everyone, but I equally think even having some device free time is good for our mental health, even if it's just having a walk in nature like I do.

Be mindful how much content online is designed to be inflammatory in nature. A quick scroll through social media can so easily ruin your mood for the day, which isn't the way to promote healing, especially since our mind and gut are so intertwined. Furthermore, social media apps are purposely designed to be addictive. Most of us overshare our every thought, and the average user is spending over four hours a day scrolling through their feeds. That's that equivalent of 60 days a year!

I was actually reading a review of a holiday resort the other day. Someone had given it a one star review because 'the WiFi wasn't very good'. You're on holiday. Nobody cares about your holiday snaps as much as you do. Stop being a slave to your device and go relax with your family.

Have a look at where you live, and see where the best walking or nature spots are. Make time to switch off once a week with your family and go get some fresh air. I promise, your GERD will thank you for it, because nature is so good for our wellbeing. Being cooped up in the same four walls all day staring at a screen isn't. Remember, we spend 90% of our time indoors, see if you can reduce that percentage as much as possible.

5.5 SOCIETAL PRESSURE

Another thing that may be causing you stress is the pressure to have everything figured out by now, or even to be the breadwinner or whatever it may be.

Somebody made a very good point about the 'fast' years of a relationship. A lot of couples get married, move in together and have kids within a very short time frame, usually between the first two to five years. This is only a small fraction of someone's entire lifespan. I wonder how many people do so, because they feel it's what's expected of them? From their family, friends and of course, society?

For some, it's going to work out beautifully. But what about those who secretly feel trapped? They have no other option because they want to make their family proud, and 'be a man' or 'provide grandchildren' etc.

People also have a problem with single people. If you're single, they try to match you up with someone, even if you're perfectly happy as you are. Any event you get invited to, you must have a plus one. They'll even pair you up with someone if you don't. Urgh!

The internal pressure we all put on ourselves can be a killer. I once read an advice column where a man wrote in feeling really stressed, because in his culture it was expected he would pay for a lavish wedding with 200 guests. He only had a minimum wage job, and was terrified he'd look 'pathetic' in front of his bride to be or family for admitting he couldn't afford the wedding. It's an extreme example I know, but this is happening and it's terrible someone should be made to feel like that.

It's also apparently a common tradition generally that an engagement ring costs 3x the man's salary. But what about the man having to pay his rent and bills? Are we actually saying the man only loves his bride to be if he makes an extreme purchase he likely cannot afford? Given an engagement ring depreciates in value as soon as you leave the shop, and half of all marriages end in divorce, isn't that the most ridiculous thing you've ever heard?

So have a think about societal stress you have personally faced. Like every example I mention in this book, it's going to be completely different for each of you. Identify anything that keeps you up at night, because ultimately it's all going to hinder not help your GERD.

Sometimes it's like peeling back an onion, where each layer is followed by another. You have to keep going to get to the crux of what is troubling you.

5.6 THE WRONG WAYS TO DEAL WITH STRESS

Continuing to ignore the warning signs your body is giving you that you are stressed is, as the above title suggests, the wrong way to deal with stress.

As we've covered, most people are diabolical at admitting they are stressed, let alone dealing with it properly. So the first thing I'd say is to admit - even just to yourself - that you need some form of a circuit breaker.

I knew in my job that I wasn't handling the stress, and in the end, I snapped. That's not the right way to do things. Equally, when there's no flexibility in the system, all you can do is get out. I hope nobody gets to the point - whatever you're stressed about - that you snap like that. Leave now while you still can. Even if it's walking away instead of getting into an argument with someone. I promise you'll feel better after some reflection, where you can come up with a more rational response.

Smoking also won't fix your stress. In practically every job I've worked at, the management are heavy smokers. They get stressed and immediately head outside for a cigarette. Now, I'm sure that relieves your stress in the *meantime*, but it's not going to have a long-lasting effect. If it did, why would you need 20 a day?

In addition, if you have GERD, smoking is one of the very worst things you can do.

Likewise, trying to eat or drink away your stress isn't going to solve the problem either. As we know, overeating with GERD or eating the wrong foods (nobody eats salad when they are stressed) is not going to help you heal.

Another aspect to avoid is taking your stress out on others. I suspect this has happened to me in the workplace on a number of occasions because when you're lower down the chain, you're an easy target, as you lack the power to challenge the person. All this does though, is spread the misery onto someone else, which eventually comes back to you when they quit their job or lodge a complaint. So whether you take your stress out on your employees, your family or the general public, whoever they may be - don't.

The Consequences Of Dealing With Stress The Wrong Way

I had the honour of being asked to edit a book for a client who had the most incredible life story.

He was a tough guy from an inner city location, the type who could take on anything, a real-life Bruce Willis hard nut, if you will. However, he went through an incredible series of traumatic events, which ranged from his father being murdered to being in a building at the precise time a helicopter crashed into it. He not only saw the immediate aftermath of that crash, but helped pull people out of the building. As a result, he developed survivor's guilt because he wasn't one of the many fatalities he'd tried to rescue. He also lost his unborn twins, among many other horrific events that just kept on coming throughout his life.

Each time something bad happened to him, his mantra was to put on his suit and tie and head to work as usual. No matter what happened, he never called in sick or even mentioned anything to his colleagues. He managed to keep up this 'stiff upper lip' act until he was involved in a car accident.

The hospital wanted to scan his head to check for injuries. So he ran out of the hospital, because he was petrified they would be able to see he was suffering from mental health problems on the scan results.

After having a breakdown and being treated for complex PTSD, he's now a mental health advocate. This man now dedicates his entire time to the cause of helping others speak out about their mental health, mostly through inspirational talks with the aim of removing the stigma of discussing mental health. Specifically, he focuses on corporate clients because he felt that the workplace was the last place where he could talk about his issues.

Now, if you just read that and you feel stressed in your life, you may dismiss your current situation because 'it's not as bad as that guy', or anyone else you can think of, especially as his issues were more trauma based rather than 'everyday' stress. Don't get me wrong, perspective can sometimes quash certain feelings and help us find a healthier way to deal with our issues. But this is not always the case, as a dismissive attitude can actually be really damaging too.

Ultimately, if you are feeling stressed because of extreme trauma or because you can't get someone to babysit - stress is stress.

The problem is as I said, we dismiss ourselves. There's always going to be someone a lot worse off than you are and those who are a lot better off. That doesn't mean what you are going through doesn't matter; it always matters. Maybe not always to those around you, but it should always matter to you. Regardless of the reasons you are stressed, all of us need to take the time to recognise it, especially if it's sustained and starting to affect our mental or physical health. If you have also experienced complex trauma, then this is even more reason to properly deal with your mental health.

As an example, going back to my client going around doing mental health talks. He's probably well aware that not everyone he will speak to will have gone through anything to the extent of what he has. That's not the point of his work. He does it to open up awareness for mental health of all kinds, big or small, that everyone goes through to some degree.

I personally think that's not only incredibly brave but so refreshing. If he'd of carried on ignoring what was going on inside his head, he'd sadly probably be yet another suicide statistic. We see this all the time.

5.7 THE RIGHT WAYS TO DEAL WITH STRESS

When you get stressed, it causes a chain reaction. You don't eat very well; you can't sleep; you begin to make mistakes at work; you get into arguments with those around you etc. We've all done it.

I don't think it's possible to never feel stress again in your life. But, we all need to get to a place where we can handle a reasonable amount of pressure and be able to diffuse a situation before it crosses an unhealthy threshold.

This may be controversial, but I think we all need to get a little more brutal in protecting our general wellbeing. We're always going to have to deal with issues and people that are difficult. But for me, it's about recognising when you've tried every alternate avenue, and you're still ending up at the same destination.

As an incredibly dull example, think about filling in a tax return. I hate doing it because I was never good at maths, and the form is incredibly long-winded and laborious. I started my last one on a Friday when I was exhausted, and I got a horrible migraine as a result that lasted for about three days. This year, I've decided to hire an accountant to go through it with me instead. Hence, I've navigated around the issue because I cannot skip reporting my tax and also because there definitely is an alternative. Even if that's just starting earlier in the week when I'm more alert.

However, the ability to find a better solution is not the case with all situations, including people you may encounter in life. Sometimes, you have to know when cutting the cord is the right thing to do, otherwise, you're going to suffer.

People may well think it's weak to walk away from a stressful situation. But, if I am in an environment where stress isn't recognised, or mental health is either mocked or ignored completely, then sometimes it's the *only option*. Yes, we'd all love it to be like a Hollywood movie where everyone bands together to overthrow the system, but the reality is we're not quite at the point where anyone is willing to do that, even if in private they tell you how much they agree with what you are saying. I know because I've had these conversations with former colleagues of my GERD-inducing job, and I can't say I blame people for being afraid when they have a lot to lose.

When we get stressed we are actually less able to be productive or creative in our work. So the first thing you need to do is concentrate on the most important task. Work your way down a list until you've taken care of everything, realising that it's physically impossible to be all things to all people.

I have a couple of ideas that will remain ideas because I know it would be impossible to get funding for. The first would be to have yearly mental health checks. It's not about trying to diagnose everyone with a problem, but rather just checking on how people are. I think it would be a great way to nip any problems in the bud and help people see if they are doing just fine or need to take a step back. I've always found it ludicrous how over the course of a lifetime, we have more checks on our teeth than we do on our mental health.

The other is that I think all towns and cities should have an open coffee shop, where people come in and chat with each other. I know this can go so badly wrong, so it would never work. But, just the idea that if you want a chat generally (especially for lonely older people), there is a designated space where that's acceptable, and you wouldn't be bothering people. Sparking conversation in general can be so good for improving mental health across the board.

In the meantime, what do we do? I think we start by realising the challenges we are going through as individuals and as the wider population. Why are we so stressed? Often, the reason has several other reasons behind it.

So, for example, an employee stressed at work because another worker didn't turn up that day. They now have to work even harder to cover them, and their performance is going to slip, and they might not get that promotion, which means they can't buy that bigger home they need for their family. It goes on and on and comes out as a massive ball of stress that isn't an easy fix. But we have to find a way.

6.0 LIFESTYLE

Our approach to lifestyle goes hand in hand with any other effort you make to heal from GERD. The problem is, most of us are overloaded with everything from work, family, toxic relationships, money worries, internet addiction, anxiety, self-esteem issues, you name it!

Think about it, though. If you don't take time to replenish your mental energy, how can you give anything 100%? Whether it's work, family or anything else you have going on, it's impossible to run on empty. So, considering your lifestyle as a whole is about addressing your needs as a human specifically.

6.1 EXERCISING WITH GERD

Exercise is a tricky subject to approach if you have acid reflux. On the one hand, exercise is one of the best things you can do to destress and lift your mood should you be feeling down or anxious. Yet, you also have to be really careful because, anatomically, you don't want to do anything that might flare up your symptoms.

What I find works best for me is to exercise first thing in the morning before eating. There was one occasion recently where I ignored my own advice, and I ate some noodles about half an hour before a pilates class. It felt like the food just got stuck, and I lost my appetite for a couple of days afterwards. I've learned my lesson.

At most, I'll eat a bowl of porridge in the morning before a mid-morning/early afternoon workout. The key is to not overfill yourself.

Having said that, it also depends on what type of exercise you do as well. Pilates or yoga requires you to contort yourself, and often this can be a real problem for your digestion. Likewise, crunches or any other moves that put your abdomen at an awkward/strained angle should be avoided. Try and keep upright as much as possible.

At the very least, I encourage walking outside, especially if you live somewhere where the weather is nice. Coastal/woodland walks are the best because they allow you to spend some much needed time in nature. If possible, leave your technology at home and just allow yourself that mental time to switch off. I know that's hard to do these days, but it's all a part of the healing process.

Whatever you do, don't eat a big meal, then go straight for a run. Unless you want your food to slosh about and the acid to fly back up with it. Be mindful of any exercises or postures that cause you an issue. You'll need to adapt your routine if so.

6.2 SLEEPING WITH GERD

You may struggle to sleep with GERD for several reasons. The most obvious point is that you don't feel very well, and this can make sleeping difficult anyway, especially if you're stressed or anxious about it.

There is nothing worse when you are unwell than not being able to sleep properly because of your symptoms. That being said, getting a good night's sleep is imperative for getting better, so it is something you need to take the time to look at.

From a GERD perspective, you should only eat light meals (especially in the evening). Try and eat at least three to four hours before going to bed so that your food has had time to start breaking down. If you eat a big meal, then immediately lie down; gravity won't keep your food (or your stomach acid) in the right place.

If you have a very stressful life, then sleeping is where you'll feel this the most. Worrying about the day ahead can wreck your sleep.

I appreciate this sounds a little 'new age hippy', but something that worked for me is listening to calming playlists before I went to sleep. Search for 'meditation music' or 'calming Buddist music', or even 'spa playlist'. Just something tranquil that, when you put your headphones on, will immediately start to calm your thoughts.

Remove technology (replace your phone with a traditional alarm clock) from the bedroom, and don't look at any screens for at least an hour before you go to bed. The reason is that the light emitted from devices sparks brain activity, which means it's on alert instead of winding down for sleep. Ensure your sleeping environment is free from clutter and generally feels relaxing to be in.

Another top tip is to sprinkle lavender oil on your pulse points or pillow before bed. If you have had a terrible sleeping pattern, I can assure you it is incredibly potent at doing the job. Lavender always puts me into an incredibly deep sleep, so I can't recommend it highly enough.

A wedge pillow is something that's specifically recommended for GERD. Or, putting books underneath the pillars of your bed on the side nearest your pillow to raise it. The idea being the angle will keep the acid from flowing back up as you sleep.

I did try the wedge pillow trick, and honestly I couldn't fall asleep on it, so it was promptly banished to the corner of my room. I have to sleep on my left side because I have thoracic outlet syndrome on my right side. I cannot fall asleep on my back naturally, and if I sleep on my right side, the circulation to my arm gets cut off. So I can only sleep on my left side, which really doesn't work with a wedge pillow. I'm a bit of a strange case here, so if you're not a light sleeper and you think it will help, you can find wedge pillows quite cheaply on Amazon.

I also want to mention that it's recommended GERD sufferers sleep on their left side anyway, as this position greatly reduces the ability for acid to flow back up.

For me, the best tip was not to eat too closely before bed time more than anything.That way, the food isn't 'sitting' in your throat - well, at least it feels that way with GERD, as you'll well know. Don't overeat either, especially if it's your last meal of the day, because the food will take longer to clear from your stomach.

In general, you want to make sure your bed is comfortable. So, think about when was the last time you got a new mattress? If it's been more than five years or you find it uncomfortable, then it's time to consider getting a new one. At the very least, a mattress topper can make a huge difference by adding cushioning and support. It's also a cheaper option than buying a new mattress if you can't afford to do so.

If you have insomnia generally, then you're going to need to identify the cause. It could be anything from too much caffeine to work stress keeping you up at night.

6.3 TRAVELLING WITH GERD

On the one hand, travel is one of the best ways to destress, meaning it could be extremely beneficial for anyone whose GERD is stress related.

However, travel in itself can be stressful and depending on where you are going to, you may be eating different foods and even at different times, which could prove awkward on your digestion. So, a bit of forward planning may be needed here if stress or diet have played a part in your GERD journey.

I've already mentioned how it's wise to take probiotics while travelling, but there are some other things to consider too.

Depending on where you are travelling to, be extra careful when it comes to things such as the quality of the drinking water. Likewise, avoid consuming raw, undercooked or potentially contaminated food. Even if you don't have GERD, you can pick up all kinds of bacteria and parasites that can cause serious gut issues, all when you might be thousands of miles away from your regular doctor and familiar healthcare system.

In 2011 I actually experienced this myself when I caught a viral bug from a group of passengers on a plane journey from London to New York. The group had been allowed on the plane despite transiting from another continent clearly very unwell. They were sitting in the row directly behind me coughing away, and I caught whatever they had. Within a day of landing in New York, I ended up having to visit the hospital with the same symptoms. It was an incredibly scary experience, and I didn't feel fully well again for quite some time after I returned home.

From that point onwards and *long before* it became fashionable, I have always carried hand sanitiser with me when I travel along with antibacterial wipes. I clean my seat on planes, along with tray tables, buckles etc., and I always use my sleeve to open doors or a piece of tissue. I can assure you that getting a nasty stomach bug on top of GERD is the very last thing you want.

Also, I know you are going away to relax, but try to make a determined effort to eat clean as much as possible. If you have GERD, you're going to need to remain careful about the types of foods and drinks that may give you a flare.

I'd also consider planning how you will manage if you do have a flare, such as consuming probiotic yoghurts or drinking camomile tea etc. If you prepare for this in advance and have everything with you that you need, then you're far less likely to encounter a problem.

Are you interested in reading about some of my GERD travel fails? If so, you're in luck.

Most of these stories relate to travelling between the UK and Los Angeles where my other half lives. It takes about 10 hours to get from LAX to LHR owing to delays in takeoff (of which there always are!) before you get to the 5,500 mile flight part. At this point in my GERD journey, I was still taking liquid antacids after eating as well as my omeprazole tablets.

All of my medication was in my case, and I felt really unwell on the flight. But I thought to myself, just ride it out. There are only a few hours until you land when you can have your next dose of medication and antacids.

When we landed, it was about 4am LA time, and I'm one of these people who can't sleep on flights anyway, let alone when I'm feeling ill. Everyone stood around the baggage carousel for about an hour, but only 20 or so bags came off the flight. It turns out Heathrow Airport had lost the others, including mine. They said they were 'somewhere in the airport and definitely here', but they couldn't tell us where. So, I had to travel three hours home on the train without my bags after not having my medication in about 12 hours at this point. Though, I was, of course, able to pick up some emergency antacid sachets at a pharmacy.

Yes, I know the wisecracks at the back will be telling me I should have packed my medication in my hand baggage. But I just had the large bottle at the time and not the smaller sachets. I'd taken my medication before I flew and never had a lost bag before. You learn these things the hard way in life.

It took them over a week to reunite me with my bags because there was a huge backlog. This then caused me more stress, and you know how stress and GERD go together. Urgh. So, learn from my mistake and always carry your medication (for whatever condition you have) with you. Yes, even if it turns out that medication doesn't really help beat your condition, because missing a dosage or suddenly stopping medication can create awful side effects.

The next time I returned to LA it was with a different airline. By this point, I'd left my job, and I was starting to get to grips with my healing, so I was able to eat some foods, but not quite everything yet.

I always check the plane menu before I travel, and as the meal looked very acidic, I opted for a 'gluten free' meal instead. I had pre-booked this in advance, the day I booked the flight.

So, of course, when it came to mealtime, they handed me a

regular meal which I knew I'd have problems eating. I asked if it was gluten free as I'd ordered, and in a sharp tone, the flight attendant said, "well, have you booked one?" I told her yes, and rolling her eyes at me, she went to go find it.

I will say for anyone with any food intolerances or dietary issues, it's nerve-wracking enough to try and sort the right food out without getting judgement from others or being treated as if you're a burden when you can't help it. I mean what are you supposed to do, eat something that may make you ill, *just* to avoid looking difficult?

Anyway, she found the meal I'd ordered sitting at the back of the plane freezing cold at this point. I remember it consisted of the smallest piece of chicken I'd ever seen in my entire life, along with about five teeny-tiny sized potatoes and gravy.

So I thought, meh okay I'll see if I can grab a snack later in the flight. Weirdly for a long haul flight, you had to pay for snacks and even the TV (this airline has gone out of business now you could probably tell that was coming). Anyway, when the snack trolley THAT YOU HAD TO PAY FOR ON A TEN HOUR FLIGHT came around, the only two choices consisted of chocolate or crisps - aka the arch-nemesis of your LES muscle and the acid it's supposed to hold in. So that was a no-go. I tried to distract myself with their 'latest blockbuster movie selection of 2018' that I'd also been fleeced for - 'You've Got Mail'. Christ sake.

They did bring a 'light meal' around four hours later, which was a lettuce sandwich on gluten-free bread that honestly tasted like soil. I also read a tweet recently that said the test for gluten intolerance should be gluten free bread because you'd never eat it otherwise. I concur.

I just had to double check that I didn't have this tab open by mistake instead of Tripadvisor there. Hang on, I'm nearly done with this story.

When I landed, my partner Isaak sensed my hangryness and drove me to this gorgeous grill place because he knew they served chicken, gravy and mashed potatoes like what I'd been eating for months on end. What a saint. But if I could do that flight again, I'd definitely pack some GERD friendly snacks with me just in case.

In general, I have to say my visits to California have been life-changing where my health is concerned, and a lot of the changes I made feature in this book.

Where I live, people head to the corner shop where you can find many processed foods like crisps (potato chips for you Americans), chocolate, fizzy drinks etc. Saturday nights are either spent getting absolutely wasted at a club or watching whatever is on TV. Sunday feels like absolute doom waiting for Monday. Rinse and repeat.

However, in California, I've found there is more of a focus on healing, self growth and getting at one with nature. Now, I know sometimes that goes into the extreme where you have the likes of Gwyneth Paltrow telling women to steam their nether regions. I don't mean all that tripe. But, I do think there's something in spending time at the beach, relaxing, drinking green smoothies etc., versus the chaotic, unhappy madness most people are stuck in. It really doesn't have to be that way, even simple changes can have a huge impact!

So if you are travelling, alongside keeping your gut healthy with probiotics, the best advice I can give is eat fresh as much as possible. Don't eat fast food or processed food, and research smoothie bars and other places where you can grab some alkaline treats, just in case the travel or change in environment results in a GERD flare. Obviously, if you are a little further on in your healing journey you can afford to loosen up a little, just don't make *really bad* dietary choices that will waste all your hard work up to now.

Also, be very weary of viruses. I know post-Covid we're *all weary* of viruses to some extent. But, they really do come in many forms, and when you're in an airport mixing with people from all over the world, you just can't be too careful where cleanliness and hygiene are concerned. In short: Don't touch things, wash your hands very often and don't eat with your hands.

6.4 EATING OUT WITH GERD

While you are healing, particularly in those early stages it's probably not a great idea to eat out, unless you plan on visiting any healthy restaurants where there's plenty of alkaline dishes on the menu. So as frustrating as it is (especially in terms of your social life) you may need to abstain for a few weeks until you feel confident to expand your palate.

The key is to continue to avoid acidic foods, greasy foods, foods high in fat along with overeating. So, only visit restaurants where you can ensure this will be the case. As restrictive as it might seem for the moment, you really don't want to offset any progress you've made up to now. There will come a time when you can stuff your face with tomatoey carbs or even a juicy burger without a care in the world. I'm living proof of this.

So think of any restaurant where the food is fried, the portions are too large, the food has an oil slick on the plate - these are the places you need to avoid for now. If the food is really bad, you may not be able to return to it because it probably makes everyone feel crap even those without GERD. Though, you could also take the opportunity to discover new restaurants you have never tried in this time. All is not lost!

Researching the menu and having a look at images of the dishes online can also be extremely helpful.

Also, watch what you drink when you eat out too. When I had GERD, I would opt for a glass of water in restaurants if they didn't have camomile tea, a green juice or a smoothie. Drinking alcohol isn't an issue in itself, but if you have GERD, alcohol or smoking is something you have to cut out. I know, it's easier said than done, but honestly if you have extremely severe symptoms it can't be as bad as carrying on as you are.

Just to recap what we've covered, even with water, it doesn't mean it's plain sailing. If they put lemon in it, then the water now has an acid in it. Which is funny because in normal circumstances, lemon water is incredibly healthy not to mention delicious. But, with GERD you may as well be squeezing it in your eyes because that's exactly what it feels like in the stomach when you drink it - see my litmus test examples.

Then there's sparkling water. I'm going to create a debate bigger than the 'correct way' to pronounce the word 'scone' here, but honestly, who decided to make water fizzy?

How about a hot chocolate, I mean that's warm and comforting right? Well, as we know chocolate contains an ingredient that loosens the LES muscle which is responsible for keeping your acid in your stomach. With GERD it feels like your LES is a saloon door in a western movie, constantly popping open in dramatic fashion with the 'gunshots' felt as hiccups. Hot chocolate also contains sugar which is inflammatory in the body. For me personally, consuming sugar causes me to have terrible skin and joint pain, so no, as much as I love the taste of it I can't have that either.

Everyone is going to have different thresholds of what they can handle. So if you find you're actually fine with any of the above, that's okay *so long as you're okay*. Like I say with everything throughout this book, listen to your body. If you have a glass of wine and it doesn't cause you symptoms, then great. What I'm saying is take it steady, and be really careful to avoid any triggers. I know it's really dull to be restricted, but you have to give your body time to heal. Otherwise this whole thing will keep on going which surely will be worse in the long run.

Oh, and if your 'friends' judge you for making the right choice for your health while you recover from GERD, meaning you can't eat out as you usually would then they aren't your actual friends. Just sayin'.

6.5 PREGNANCY AND GERD

Yet another disclaimer here is that I'm not a doctor. Nor have I ever been pregnant. However, pregnancy and GERD are often two things that go hand in hand. I was actually watching a video on YouTube the other day where an American OBGYN was talking about pregnant patients who suffer from heartburn or long term GERD. Her explanation was that the hormones released in pregnancy loosen up the muscles, including the LES muscle, and if so, this can produce some of the symptoms associated with old wives' tales of 'the baby growing hair'.

Normally, the LES muscle acts as a doorway keeping your stomach acid firmly contained. But hormones can disrupt this, making the door essentially pop open and stay that way either for short periods or sometimes longer. Often, pregnancy related GERD will go away on its own, but it can be incredibly bothersome while you are going through it.

Having suffered severely with GERD, I can only imagine how difficult it must be to have it while pregnant too. Not only is your body going through lots of changes, but you're also trying to grow a human inside of you. Not being able to eat properly during that time must be incredibly difficult, so kudos to anyone experiencing this right now.

I encourage you to speak to your doctor about your symptoms. I say this because GERD is so commonly associated with pregnancy, meaning it's easy to accept it as 'part and parcel' of what you should expect. But, if it's at the point where you are *really* struggling and becoming quite weak, then you need to consult with the right people. As always, I do suggest a nice hot cup of camomile tea to see if this settles anything.

(Though I haven't found anything to suggest camomile is harmful, not all teas are recommended for pregnant women, so please seek medical clearance before you eat or drink anything new if you are unsure).

As a final note, I will say all the rules and regulations surrounding what you should and shouldn't do during pregnancy seems highly stressful in itself. I get it; we all want to be safe, of course, we do. But, I think we are at such an extreme level that it's doing more harm than good. We know that you shouldn't drink alcohol during pregnancy; that's a complete given. But, the list of what you should avoid goes into such extreme detail that I genuinely think it's frightening women. Even some beauty products are labelled as not suitable for pregnant women. Where does it end?

While you should 100% follow official guidance, be sure to watch your stress levels in the process because that's the silent harm nobody is talking about. Like the women who had a glass of wine not realising they were in the early stages of pregnancy and continue to beat themselves up about it even after the baby is born perfectly healthy. Only, there's nothing you can do, you cannot take it back and more to the point, you didn't do it deliberately. Yet, for some women, it can really lead to guilt and shame, thinking they are a 'bad parent'. When, surely the definition of a 'bad parent' is someone who doesn't care at all?

If you are pregnant and currently highly anxious about every little thing, please remember to breathe. You are doing the best you possibly can, and that's all anyone can ask of you. It will also really help your GERD if you reduce your stress levels too.

At the end of the day, your baby matters but so do you, so please don't suffer in silence with any symptoms you are going through, least of all GERD. The good news is that unlike ever exploding nappies (diapers, if you will) - GERD is something you can recover from.

6.6 POSTURE AND GERD

When was the last time you thought about your skeleton? Namely, I'm talking about your ribcage and all of the organs, including your digestive system that is stored within it. Far too many of us have crap posture these days, especially if you spend time slumped over your computer or looking down at your phone.

You might not think posture is a big deal, but what if your car wheels didn't sit in the right place, or the bricks of your home weren't lined up correctly? At some point, you'd run into a problem. GERD is just one of the many, many ailments that can arise due to poor posture. So now is the time to listen to your granny, who always told you to 'stand up straight'. Well, mine used to ask if I had a tenner to buy a bottle of whisky but you know what I mean.

I make time every day to work on my posture through stretching and two pilates classes each week. Even still, such efforts are pointless if you don't actively throw those shoulders back and keep yourself in a good alignment throughout the day.

If you're not sure, look at yourself in the mirror as you work and check your posture. Better still, get a posture assessment to see if anything is off balance. Doing so might just help you avoid other health problems in the future, too, including joint and disc problems.

6.7 LIFESTYLE TOP TIPS

Be sure to check in with your dentist if you've been experiencing long term GERD. I was actually writing the website content for a client of mine, and in there, I had to mention how GERD can affect your teeth. Then I remembered I, too, suffered from GERD and thought ah crap.

Stomach acid has a pH of anywhere between 1.5 and 3.5, whereas dental enamel begins to erode at pH 5.5. Remember, acidic is classed as anything from a pH 0 to around pH 6.0. So you definitely don't want stomach acid on your teeth, especially not for years due to GERD.

Again, I'm not mentioning this to scare you because if you've been through GERD, then you've suffered enough. But, you do need to be aware that acid flying out where it's not supposed to be can cause issues for wherever it lands. So in the esophagus, we know it can irritate the lining, cause pain, scarring etc. In the voicebox, it can cause people to sound hoarse for weeks. When stomach acid hits the teeth, it can cause problems with your enamel because the two are never supposed to actually meet.

So, as well as doing everything you can to heal yourself, I would certainly check in with your dentist and just let them know what's been happening. I've personally been ok at dental checkups, but I'd still rather everyone reading this just know it's something to look out for rather than not be given any advice at all. In addition, following diligent dental hygiene is going to help you out in this regard.

Toothpaste And GERD

This is a bit of a weird one, but you may notice certain toothpastes and mouthwashes seriously flare up your GERD. After all, mint is terrible for GERD, so when you think about it, this makes sense.

Of course, you can't not brush your teeth. Where possible, I'd recommend ditching ultra minty toothpastes until you recover. I'm personally not a fan of flavoured toothpaste, but some of you might get on well with it.

When you brush, take care not to swallow any toothpaste at all. Rinse your teeth really well, once if not twice, with water for about 30 seconds. It might seem like overkill, but if there's any trace of mint in your mouth, the vapours may trigger the acid to come up.

This leads me nicely to mouthwash. Again, use mouthwash but avoid letting it too near the back of your throat (I know, this sounds more like I'm training you to join the circus). Don't use mouthwashes that contain alcohol, and again avoid super minty ones.

When I was at my worst, even the smell of mouthwash on other people as they spoke near me would bring acid into my throat. So, if this has happened to you, you're not alone. At least now you can be aware of the issue and ditch the mint until you feel better.

Since I've recovered, the mint hasn't bothered me, though I still avoid mouthwashes that contain alcohol. Mostly because they make me feel like I've had a chemical burn, but I digress.

Tight Clothing

If you want to promote better digestion, then tight clothing ain't it. I'm talking specifically about tight clothing that covers your abdomen, from tight trousers to tight t-shirts. Even belts that are done up too tightly - you get the idea.

For anyone who wears a bra, make sure it isn't too tight either. It's actually a fact that 90% of women wear the wrong bra size. It's recommended to get a bra fitting every six months, or after you've lost or gained weight. If your bra is too tight around your chest, it can compress everything that's already upset with you digestion wise, which will only make things worse.

I'm a huge fan of 'cami style' bras with wide straps. You can even find tank top style bras that are incredibly supportive without an underwire. If yours is digging into you as you read this, go sort it out!

Non-bra wearers: Sorry you had to read all that but honestly, just be thankful you don't get to the end of the day and feel as if you've had a wooden shelf attached to your chest all day (underwired bras).

Screens

The latest statistics suggest that Americans check their phones at an average of every four minutes, which equates to 360 times a day.

You might not be American reading this nor your phone usage as extreme, but it's fair to say we all spend a bit too much time immersed in screens, meaning, like our devices, we never really switch off properly.

Technology is here to stay, and our lives are better in many ways for it. But when it comes to your mental health in particular and the health of your relationships, you also need to know where the balance lies. So, if you're someone who goes on a date and spends the whole time scrolling through social media and basically cannot go a few minutes without tapping that screen, you're probably not as focused on your healing, let alone your wellbeing as a whole as you should be.

Exposure to screens also messes with our circadian rhythm and can be extremely disruptive to sleep, which is essential for our health too. If you're not sleeping probably, your body isn't getting an adequate chance to replenish, and you may turn to unhealthier foods and habits just to get through the next day. It soon becomes a slippery slope.

So while it's not always possible to ditch your phone altogether, it's good to remember that *true* health and happiness can never be found within likes, shares, followers or retweets. If your phone is actually producing constant alerts and notifications, then it's probably causing you more stress than you might realise. Is there anything you can do to strike a better balance from this point on?

7.0 THE POST GERD YEARS

I'm at a stage now where I can eat most foods, bar anything extremely fatty such as deep fried foods. I never ate fried foods *that* often before, but now they are a definite no-no.

But by and large, my eating is mostly back to normal. I can indulge on the weekends, so long as I avoid the super greasy stuff. I always follow up with probiotics and camomile tea.

To destress I now do pilates and yoga every single day. Just for context I have never done yoga in my life, and I was about as flexible as a lamppost before I started. I'm a few months in now and I'm now starting to get it.

I will say I have continued to experience flashbacks to my old job and perpetual self doubt about my ability as a writer.

Though, recently I had a breakthrough on that front. I attended an online writing master class by the utterly brilliant Jay Rayner, who is a British journalist known for his restaurant reviews. This is probably the third time I've mentioned him in this book now - soz.

Anyway, I asked him a question about overcoming criticism within a newsroom environment to the level I did, and in particular with my boss.

In that moment, Jay could have quite easily told me it's part and parcel of what to expect as a writer. After all, he edited his first newspaper before I was even born and now he writes for the nationals. But no, he called that behaviour out and told me and others in so many words to keep on writing. It was one of the most inspiring interactions I've ever had with someone.

Yes, childishly I did play the clip where he went on to call my boss an 'arsehole' about 20 times on repeat before I went to bed that night. On Twitter, other attendees were quoting him saying they had experienced something similar. Unbelievably, when I clicked on a couple of their profiles, they only worked for the exact same newsgroup! Then you realise this sort of stuff isn't in your head as they want you to believe, it's widespread.

When someone you look up to you instils confidence in you, it's life-changing. So if you, like me, had any mental health related caused behind your GERD, I hope you find a similar level of closure, even if it's the ability to never look back at a situation that caused your body to literally attack itself with its own acid.

It's not about having a fragile ego either. Like I said, we all have to be able to take criticism, and in many ways it's the only way to become better. But there's a line you don't cross, especially when at the end of the day you're supposed to be a team. It makes no sense to me when leaders turn on the ones they are supposed to be setting an example to. I wanted to learn from them and be the best I could, instead their treatment coupled with the lack of support for what the job actually entailed left me feeling like a shell of myself. No wonder the industry has such a high turnover rate. This cannot be incidental.

7.1 WHAT I WOULD HAVE TOLD MYSELF

I made it this far in the book without quoting a hero of mine, Tori Amos. She has a song called Crucify, which I think is apt for how we all push on with GERD instead of addressing the issue as we should. The exact lines of the song I'm thinking of here is, "Why do we crucify ourselves every day? I crucify myself, and nothing I do is good enough for you."

The underlying question here is, *why* do we do it? Why do we all push ourselves harder than we should, even when our bodies are screaming at us? Why do we put up with crappy work conditions that make us miserable, despite the fact we go above and beyond to please people who lack the ability to be pleased in the first place? Why do we eat foods that are more like chemical experiments rather than address our feelings?

Because we *think* we don't have a choice. But like I said earlier on, if there's a door, then there's always a choice. So what are you going to choose? I choose health.

7.2 WHAT I WANT HEALTHCARE PROFESSIONALS TO KNOW

Anyone reading this related to the healthcare profession, particularly in the treatment of GERD, I think it's commendable you are doing so much research about the condition by reading this book, especially when I'm a patient and not a fellow professional.

You don't need me to tell you we have a big problem on our hands where GERD is concerned, given it is one of the most common health conditions that also happens to be both poorly understood and managed. I'm also acutely aware that healthcare facilities around the world are either stretched or not accessible enough. Especially post-pandemic.

That said, I want every doctor's office in the world to offer free information for patients about the causes of acid reflux, along with foods they should and should not eat. Even if you have to create a page on your website or produce a leaflet, please, at the very least, give people a background of what is causing their condition and how they can get better.

If you send them away with tablets or antacids with no dialogue, that's not going to help your patients get to the root cause of their problems. But if you have such resources to hand, where you can give them further reading, it's going to help people in the long term.

I know that med school directs you to medication. But, the best medication ultimately is overhauling your diet and lifestyle. Of course, you're not just going to stop prescribing medication to people, I get it, and that's not what I'm directly saying.

However, I do think collectively, healthcare providers and governments need to work to steer people in the right direction. It's difficult because people don't want to be told what to do. But ultimately, if we want to 'save the NHS' and reduce pressures on healthcare systems around the world, we have to become healthier, so we all use the services less.

Believe me; I do not want to be clogging up your diary with endless appointments where I feel like I'm not getting anywhere, and neither do the vast majority of your patients, I'm sure. But that's what will continue to happen if the advice and treatment options don't directly target the causes of problems.

I'm sure for many doctors, you feel frustrated. I would be more than happy to help any medical professional or provider with help and advice from a patient's perspective. Or maybe, you could school your own patients to try and figure out a more effective way to reach a solution. If there is any way we can work to improve the experience for other patients, then I'm all for it. Though hopefully, you've got what you needed from this book.

8.0 CONCLUSION

Firstly, thank you for purchasing and reading my book and getting to the conclusion. Alternatively, if you've opened this last page first because you thought there was an easy way out of GERD haha try again, son.

In all seriousness, my sincere hope is that you reach the closing segment of this book and feel confident in knowing how to manage your GERD. The simplest way to describe the transformation is getting in tune with what your body needs of you, rather than working against it.

Anytime you get a flare-up of GERD, whether the symptoms are mild or more severe, it's an indicator that something isn't quite agreeing with your body. While it's certainly unpleasant to go through, it's your opportunity to do something about it by listening and reacting in all the right ways we have discussed.

As I have stressed, there's no specific time frame in which you will heal, and you will have good and bad days. But, at least you have the company of a former GERD patient to guide you through, so I hope this has and will continue to offer you some comfort.

5 Reasons Why You May Struggle To Recover From GERD

I'm not a doctor nor a miracle worker, nor am I responsible for your healing. That said, I want every single person to get to the bottom of their GERD and create meaningful changes that are going to help them.

So if things aren't going to plan, here are five reasons in no particular order I think would make the best starting points to get you back on track. Some are going to need to be discussed with your doctor, and others you may be able to work on yourself.

You Don't Have GERD

Could it be you've been misdiagnosed? If you refresh yourself with the GERD symptoms at the start of this book, you should notice an overlap with what you are experiencing. For example, a burning feeling in the chest, bringing acid up into the throat, difficulty swallowing, pain when eating acidic foods or drinks etc.

These symptoms could also not be GERD because so many difficult medical conditions exist. So, if you've given it everything and enough time has passed, go back for a second opinion. Write all of your symptoms down so that your doctor won't miss any clues. Tell them what you've been trying and whether it's helped or not.

Your GERD Triggers Haven't Been Identified

GERD can be caused by many different things, including diet, general eating habits, stress, anxiety, hormonal changes or anatomical defects.

You may not be fully aware of all of your triggers, meaning you could be doing things that are causing a flare-up without you realising. If so, it's time to recap on the causes of GERD to try and eliminate your personal triggers.

You Need More Tests

When a problem with the stomach, the stomach acid or the LES valve is detected, it's not always a simple fix.

You may need to return to a doctor or a specialist for more in-depth testing so that your treatment will be more effective.

You Haven't Given It Enough Time

Even when you are doing all of the right things, you can't expect to heal from a chronic condition overnight. It personally took me around six months to feel good again after a year of my symptoms being out of control.

Time is relative to each person, but even probiotics can take a few weeks to work. If you are following every step and you've ruled out other conditions (i.e. you know you're on the right path), you should start to feel better within a few weeks.

Eating the wrong foods or partaking in activities that we know trigger GERD will set your recovery back. So, it's important you give it all you've got and really concentrate on healing before deciding you can't be bothered to see it through. I know this won't be most of you who are trying, but just to cover all bases here, use your common sense. If you're feeling at least somewhat better, continue and be patient.

You Aren't Fully Listening To All The Information

There is so much to absorb with GERD and digestive health in general that it's easy to miss key pieces of information. I don't think there's more I could have told you in this book, as I've strived to be as comprehensive as is possible for a patient and not a doctor, at least.

That said, it's always worth making the effort to do your research. Think about anything that doesn't make your stomach feel so good or habits that you notice induce your symptoms. These could well be GERD triggers you weren't even aware of. Don't be too hard on yourself, but do make an effort to inform yourself, and most of all, listen to what your own body is telling you about how you are treating it.

GERD Recovery Checklist

- I have seen a doctor and reported all of my symptoms to rule out any other conditions
- I know the underlying cause(s) of my GERD so that I know how to address my symptoms
- While I recover, I am not eating high fat foods, processed foods, acidic foods, smoking, drinking alcohol, drinking coffee or taking drugs to ensure my GERD will not be triggered by these activities
- I am not eating at least three to four hours before bed after my evening meal
- I am not overeating, and I am ensuring I take the time to eat my food properly so as to not inhibit my digestion
- I am taking probiotics daily along with any supplements my doctor has recommended to support my nutrition
- I am exercising but not in a way that will strain my digestive system physically
- I am actively making time each day to look after my mental health and wellbeing
- I am committed to taking the steps which are helping me to heal for as long as necessary, and I take full responsibility for my own healing journey
- I will seek medical help if at any time I develop new or usual symptoms that were not present prior to my last medical checkup
- After I have healed, I will make a continued effort to look after my health as a whole and will not return to any damaging habits I know directly attributed to my GERD because I do not want to end up back here
- I will seek further help and support if I feel unable to stop any behaviours or activities or which are resulting in my symptoms

8.1 GERD FAQ

For those in need of some quickfire answers, I thought a GERD FAQ would be most helpful.

Now, if you've read this book in its entirety, you will notice I have already covered each of these topics in great depth, so I'd suggest going back and reading the applicable section.

However, if you're in search of a concise answer, this is designed to give you a brief overview of what I have experienced as a patient, along with the research I have carried out to write this book.

Once again for the folks at the back, it is **not** a substitute for a medical checkup.

What Causes Acid Reflux?

Acid reflux can occur for a wide variety of reasons, including due to stress, anxiety, diet, general eating habits, obesity, pregnancy, anatomical defects of the digestive system or smoking.

In short, in the vast majority of cases, we stress our digestive system with acidic habits or a lifestyle that is not compatible with our own human needs.

That's why before moving forward with a healing strategy, you identify your personal GERD triggers. As mentioned, my GERD was primarily caused by stress, though diet and my general eating habits also played a part.

How Is GERD Diagnosed?

It's possible to recognise symptoms of GERD in yourself by looking at what you are experiencing and matching this up with what the symptoms are, along with how other patients such as myself have described how they felt physically. For example, burning in the chest, an inability to swallow, a painful dry stomach etc.

Then what you need to do is go to the doctor with all of this information, who will look to rule out any other causes such as a heart problem (for those with shortness of breath), appendicitis (for those with pain on one side) etc.

Depending on your symptoms, they may run further tests to rule these conditions out or explore your GERD in further depth. Usually, once they suspect GERD or even heartburn, you'll be given medication and sent on your way. Hence, how you probably ended up here!

Is GERD Curable?

Yes. I've made a grave error with this book title if not! I do believe that if you identify the causes of your GERD and give your healing everything you've got based on your personal triggers, you'll make huge improvements.

I would consider myself 95% back to normal, with that 5% taking into account how our stomach acid depletes as we age, meaning even if you've never had GERD, overindulging as you start to get a bit older isn't going to feel great for *anyone*.

I am at the stage where I rarely get any GERD flare-ups unless I've had an extremely stressful event or I've eaten something at a restaurant that I didn't realise was going to be *super* greasy until I started eating it (I can handle mild grease fine). I can eat most foods without issue - even treat foods that aren't the healthiest, especially if I eat these earlier in the day, bearing in mind the quality of stomach acid can also deplete throughout the day.

I enjoy the odd bit of junk food and, of course, chocolate. I eat spicy foods as well as a wide variety of foods. I also drink my own body weight in coffee.

But, I also listen to my gut, and if anything even slightly makes me feel ill, I stop. I also actively look to avoid ultra processed and basically nasty foods wherever possible, just out of personal preference because they don't nourish you.

Even when there have been times when I've had minor setbacks, I know how to immediately remedy the situation, so I've never been even close to how badly ill I was. I can usually bring my symptoms back under control within a matter of hours, bearing in mind I probably have less than five bad days a year now. Restaurant menus are finally exciting again.

What Are The Symptoms Of GERD In Adults?

Symptoms of GERD can be extremely varied and will differ from person to person. The most common symptoms include a burning sensation in the chest, chest pain, difficulty swallowing, sensation of a lump in the throat, shortness of breath, sore throat and general heartburn symptoms. These are the most common symptoms but are not exhaustive.

Can GERD Cause Shortness Of Breath?

Yes, shortness of breath is a common GERD side effect. However, due to the nature of this symptom potentially being any number of conditions, including cardiac related, you need to get all of the sinister things ruled out first before you start treating it as GERD.

Which Side To Sleep On With GERD?

The left, as this will mean your stomach will remain lower than the esophagus, making it much more difficult for the acid to flow back up. Combined with not eating three to four hours before bed, you should really notice a difference in comfort.

How Long Does GERD Take To Heal?

There is no definite answer to how long a person will take to heal from GERD. The time frame is going to depend on your cause of GERD, whether you identify all of your triggers, the techniques you use to heal and whether you commit to what you need to do or if you fall into any bad habits again. Even when you're doing all the right things, it may take some weeks to start to feel better and months if your GERD is extremely severe, as was the case for me.

Also, there are no quick fixes or overnight cures for GERD. It's a process because it's a chronic problem. Go back to your doctor if you notice any new or unusual symptoms, but otherwise, you'll need to stick with the healing strategy.

What Foods Should Be Avoided With GERD?

Foods that are processed, fried, high in fat or acidic (including healthy acidic foods such as tomatoes, lemons or spicy food). Also sodas, coffee and alcohol (especially spirits).

You also need to ditch anything you've personally found to be a trigger, regardless of whether it's on the official list or not. The question is, how does that food make **YOU** feel? Listen to your body.

Can GERD Cause Diarrhoea And Vomiting?

While I mentioned GERD can have a wide range of symptoms, diarrhoea and vomiting aren't typically associated with GERD as far as I'm aware. I think these types of symptoms point more to a viral infection or another digestive complaint, so please speak to a doctor if your symptoms either persist or don't seem to fit with GERD so that you get the right help.

8.2 GERD BE GONE

Finally, I am unable to personally respond to each message I receive. However, I have created a free resource for ongoing GERD support and information, which you can find at www.gerdbegone.com.

Part of the reason for creating this website is that my YouTube channel was originally a beauty channel, and the response to the original video I made on my GERD struggles was so acute that I wanted to create a single point of access for people to learn more. The purchase of this book will also support the site fees and time taken out of my own work to write content and maintain the website.

If you have any stories you'd be happy to be featured on my website or have any wellbeing products that may be useful to my audience, please use the contact form on the website, and if it's something I can use, I will be in touch.

ABOUT THE AUTHOR

The Rachael Edit

Rachael is a writer and YouTuber who went through a severe period of GERD in her late twenties. After posting a video about her struggles on her channel and receiving thousands of comments with people around the world all going through the same thing, she became determined to help others to recover. Sharing her experiences of GERD from a patient's perspective, Rachael aims to guide fellow patients to identify causes of their symptoms and ultimately take ownership of their health from this point onwards.

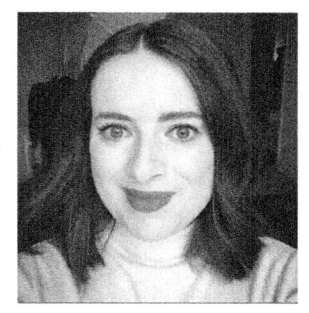

Printed in Great Britain
by Amazon

17601656R00149